DISCOVER

YOUR BEST

KETO NOW

DISCLAIMER

While every precaution is taken in preparation of this book, the publisher and author assume no responsibility for errors, omissions, contrary interpretations on the subject matter or for damages resulting from the use of the information contained herein.

This book is supplied at your individual request for information purposes only. The author is neither a doctor nor a nutritionist. No medical or nutritional advice is given. This material does not replace the advice of your doctor or qualified healthcare professional.

No guarantees on or promises for weight loss, diet, health, products, or other results—of any kind—are being made by the author or publisher, and no liabilities are being assumed. The reader is entirely responsible for his or her own actions.

Consult your doctor before starting any diet or exercise regimen.

FOLLOW AUTHOR

Connect with or follow author at:

Email: mike@letsketonow.com

Blog: https://www.letsketonow.com

https://www.pinterest.com/discoverketo/

https://twitter.com/mikewessels5

Join other fans of Discover Your Best Keto Now community by joining the FREE author-led Facebook group: Discover Your Best Keto Now:
https://www.facebook.com/groups/172968950657202/

DISCOVER

YOUR BEST

KETO NOW

Step-by-Step Weight Loss Guide

Mike Wessels

Smart Beginners Series Book 1

DEDICATION

I dedicate this book to my wife, Cindy, for her constant support and encouragement during my Keto diet and during the writing of this book.

I also dedicate this book to all my readers who struggle with weight loss. Like you, I have struggled with weight loss for over 40 years, experiencing the diet roller coaster first hand.

CONTENTS

STEP 1
LEARN THE KETO PROCESS

Ketogenic Diet

    Standard Keto Diet (SKD)

    Cyclical Keto Diet (CKD)

    High Protein Keto Diet (HPKD)

    Targeted Keto Diet (TKD)

    Advantages & Disadvantages of Keto

How Keto Works

    Glucose

    Ketones

    High Carb Diet

    Low Carb Diet

Ketosis

    Ketone Zone

    Crossing the Ketosis Barrier

    Nutritional Ketosis

    Optimal Ketosis

    Post Exercise Ketosis

    Starvation Ketosis

    Ketoacidosis

    Getting Kicked Out of Ketosis

    Keto Testing

The Ketogenic Diet

The Ketogenic diet (a.k.a. Keto) is a low carbohydrate (carbs), high fat, moderate protein diet. After reading this book, you decide if Keto is right for you. For me, Keto was and still is my best choice.

Many books are published about Keto, which may make it confusing because each author's take on this diet is different. Every dieter who has tried Keto may provide their own brand of advice and personal experience. As you read this book, I provide my own take from my personal experience on Keto. I also provide summaries from books, blogs, and research articles to synthesize and rationalize information in the following chapters and subsections.

Keto provides some guidelines. It can be confusing at times because it seems to contradict itself, but you can mold this diet into your own special diet to meet your expectations, schedule, or weight loss demands. The Keto diet offers four varieties:

- Standard Keto Diet (SKD)

- Cyclical Keto Diet (CKD)

- High Protein Keto Diet (HPKD)

- Targeted Keto Diet (TKD)

I have tried each of these Keto diets. I recount my personal experience to give you inspiration and hope because my philosophy is—as the old clique goes—*if I can do it, you can do it.*

Standard Keto Diet (SKD)

The SKD is a low-carb, moderate protein, and high fat diet. However, dieters have divided this diet into two SKD subtypes: A low carb diet and a very low carb diet (Mawer, 2018). The difference is that the very low carb diet restricts the daily carb intake to less than 20 grams (g) daily, while the low carb typically restricts carbs from about 30 to 50 grams daily, to even as high as 75 to 100 grams daily. The less strict Keto compares to the Atkins and the Paleo Diets.

After a week, most dieter's body moves into a state of nutritional ketosis. Nutritional ketosis is a metabolic state that the body is burning ketones instead of glucose as a primary fuel source (Villines, 2019). See the Ketosis chapter for more information.

The typical ratio for the SKD diet is as follows:

75% Fat, 20% Protein, 5% Carbs

To calculate this ratio into grams and calories, carbs and protein contribute 4 calories per gram, and fat contributes 9 calories per gram. If you're consuming 1600 calories (kcal) per day, to make this ratio work you must eat the following calories and grams:

1200 kcal Fat, 320 kcal Protein, 80 kcal Carbs

or

133 grams (g) Fat, 80 g Protein, 20 g Carbs or less

The SKD provides flexibility to change the above ratio to suit a busy schedule, an unorthodox diet arrangement, or any restrictive diet schedule and still lose weight from the most stubborn areas of the body (Villines, 2019).

Cyclical Keto Diet (CKD)

The CKD is like the SKD; however, the dieter follows the standard Keto for five days, and then for one to two days, eats higher intake of carbs. The one- or two-day stretch each week allows the dieter to turn the ratio on its ear, while eating 50 to 100 g of carbs each day (Rodal, 2019). If you follow some of the Hollywood celebrities or athletes, you'll find they follow this cyclical diet and maintain a demanding weight size.

Most carbs come from vegetables and fruit rather than from bread, pasta, or rice. Smart beginners may follow this diet after they have been dieting for one or two months.

This diet may not be for everyone. This diet may not be for anyone with type 2 diabetes without close glucose monitoring; however, this diet may be good for those who are resetting their metabolism or maintaining a specific weight.

This diet may fit the food consumption demands and rigorous workout routine of athletes and body builders. It's recommended the smart beginners space these two days apart from each other. Try not to consume high carbs on back-to-back days.

High Protein Keto Diet (HPKD)

The HPKD is like CKD. This diet is also for athletes and body builders, who require higher concentration of protein. The advantages of HPKD are the energy gained from protein. The disadvantages are that the body can convert protein into glucose. Therefore, dieters who are not actively working out 3 to 8 hours daily, 5 to 7 days a week find this diet may kick them out of ketosis because of the extra glucose from protein (Gunnars, 2018).

If you are consuming more than the SKD ratio in protein without exercising, you may also gain weight. Smart beginners or seasoned pros do not consider HPKD as part of their ketogenic diet because Keto is not a high protein consumption diet.

I don't recommend this diet for anyone who has type 2 diabetes unless you are rigorously exercising. You determine for yourself if this diet is for you.

Targeted Keto Diet (TKD)

The TKD is like the SKD, except for eating more carbs when you work out. Therefore, dieters, who are actively working out will consume more carbs on their regularly scheduled days before their work out times. If you plan to lose weight while on this diet, only consume extra calories from the carbs on days when you plan to work out or be very active. Be sure to calculate the calories and carbs consumed into your total calorie and carb count for the day.

Like CKD, it's recommended to eat carbs from vegetables and fruit rather than from bread, pasta, or rice.

I recommend smart beginners consume no more than 50 g of carbs on the workout days unless you are performing cardio, karate, judo, or any of the other strenuous exercise to increase the heart rate to 146 beats per minute.

Before starting any of these ketogenic diets and exercise, it's recommended to consult and receive a physical examination from your personal doctor or healthcare provider.

Advantages of Keto

The advantages of a Keto diet are inspiring. This diet gives those who follow it hope to regain their health and to live a healthier lifestyle (Gunnars, 2018).

- Lowers blood sugar. Prevents and reverses pre-diabetes and type 2 diabetes. Eliminates the need for insulin and insulin injections

- Reduces hunger and eliminates hunger cravings between meals, allowing greater success with fasting

- Feel fuller faster than with a low-fat diet and reduces the urge of overeating

- Lose fat faster. The body burns fat faster when in the state of nutritional and optimal ketosis opposed to burning glucose

- Reduces or eliminates high blood pressure

- Lowers Triglyceride levels

- Improves HDL (the good) cholesterol even though exercise is still needed

- Lowers LDL (the bad) cholesterol

- Prevents various cancers and reduces cancer growth. Cancer cells require large amounts of glucose to reproduce at rapid rates, and these cells cannot use ketones; therefore, cancer cells' reproductive rate is stifled while the body is in ketosis (Satterthwaite, 2018).

- Treats Epilepsy, Alzheimer's, Parkinson's though medical scientist are still researching the connection between these diseases and Keto (Kossoff, 2017)

- Improves memory

- Reduces or eliminates chronic systemic inflammation. The Keto diet contains anti-inflammatory effects because the body as a whole relies on glucose to become inflamed. When the glucose supply runs short, the body puts inflammation and other ailments on hold. The good part of inflammation, which is the body's ability to heal is not affected by a low carb diet

- Improves heart health

- Minimizes muscle loss even when the calorie intake is decreased

- Improves exercise performance. After adapting to ketosis, you experience higher athletic performance

Disadvantages of Keto

- **Fatigue**: After restricting carbs from your body's energy process, your body must start using ketones. Because of the fatigue, your body is going through the symptoms of withdrawal from glucose. The fatigue may be a welcomed symptom of crossing into ketosis. Once you are in ketosis, the feeling of fatigue is replaced by the abundance of energy, signifying your body's successful transition to ketosis

- **Headache**: Like the fatigue symptom, your body starts using ketones. The headache is another welcomed symptom of ketosis. Once you are in ketosis, the headaches disappear

- **Bad breath**: Bad breath is a result of an enzyme being produced during ketosis (Musa-Veloso, Likhodii, Cunnane, 2002, 65-70). The day that my wife told me I had bad breath, I was happy because I knew my body was now a fat burning machine

- **Smelly urine**: If you have a sensitive nose, you may smell a strong stench from your urine. It means your body is in nutritional or optimum ketosis

How Keto Works

Imagine your body's storage system as fuel tanks (a.k.a. the body's store). These storage tanks consist of three food groups: Carbohydrates (carbs), Fat, and Protein.

Most people consume approximately 225 grams or more daily in carbs on a 2000-calorie diet (Gunnars, 2018). I assume most of these carbs are from bread, pasta, and rice. These foods have been our daily staples since moving out of our cave dwelling times.

However, if overly consumed, these staples lead to diseases such as diabetes, heart disease, high blood pressure, high cholesterol, high triglycerides, and even cancer (Holland, 2019). As a child and young adult, I was told this condition was hereditary and irreversible, and the only way to combat these diseases was through portion control and exercise. Not true.

If you learn how to manipulate the food groups, the body will burn fat better than it burned glucose.

Glucose

Before starting a ketogenic diet, my body burned glucose for fuel because glucose is easy for my body to attain and easy to make. Like all properties of science, the body creates fuel through the path of least resistance or manipulation. Glucose is easier for the body to obtain and consume or burn as fuel; however, glucose is not an efficient fuel for the body because it needs insulin to help the body consume it, and then the body must continue to re-fuel often. This refueling causes highs and lows or insulin spikes. Therefore, to re-fuel, the body sends messages to the brain such as cravings to acquire more glucose raw materials such as sugar, simple sugars, and carbohydrates (Satterthwaite, 2018).

Ketones

Ketones are an enzyme that the body creates from the liver using stored fat (Paoli, Bosco, Camporesi, Mangar, 2015). Ketones are a better source of fuel than glucose; however, the body must exert more effort to create ketones than it does to create glucose.

A common science factor is that science takes the path of least resistance or effort. Therefore, the body chooses to make glucose because it's easier. The body takes all fats consumed and stores them until it runs low or out of glucose.

Then the brain sends messages in the form of food cravings to eat more glucose making raw materials such as carbs and simple sugars. When the body stops making glucose, the body must start burning stored fat. The burning of stored fat is how to turn your body into a fat-burning machine. I will explain this further in the Ketosis section. For now, look at how nature keeps you from starving to death.

Because of this fat storage system, nature protects you from dying of starvation. Thousands of years ago, when people were cave dwellers and hunters of food, people hunt food by chasing down prey, wrestling it to the ground, and killing it for food. These hunters and their families had to exist for days between meals or die of starvation. When these hunters were successful, they and their families gorged themselves on meat, animal fat, grains, fruit, and other carbohydrates. Their bodies stored these carbohydrates as fats for days of famine. When the hunters ran out of food or when hunting became scarce, their bodies protected them from starving to death by producing ketones from their livers as a fuel source. These hunters and their families burned the stored fat for fuel until their next kill.

Fast forward to today, people no longer hunts for food because of the ease of raising and trading food. Big box stores and big grocery store chains make the availability of food easier today than any time in human history. Unfortunately, this availability rushes in a new era and a new medical and physical condition known today as obesity, diabetes, and heart disease.

However, by following a ketogenic diet, you are forcing your body to stop burning glucose as fuel and start burning stored fat as fuel. The body must produce ketones to convert the stored fat into fuel. Ketones become a better, more efficient fuel source than glucose.

High Carb Diet

In a nutshell, you consume high carbs, making the glucose level rise. The pancreas secrets insulin. The insulin takes the glucose into the cells, providing energy to the cells.

Most people are unaware of how much they consume, especially of carbs. It is estimated that people consume between 225 grams or more carbs per 2000 calorie diet daily. If the body burns 30 grams to 50 grams per 2000 calorie diet per day, what happens to the rest of these grams?

The body doesn't waste resources, and it first converts these carbs into a complex molecule known as triglycerides and neatly stores them as fat. Most fat is stored on the body in the belly area, while other fats are stored in the arms, legs, back, shoulders, or any other available place.

When the body's carb storage system runs low, it triggers symptoms of hunger and cravings to refill the carb tank. These symptoms can be slight or massive depending on the food type and the hunger.

If the dieter is trying to get past these symptoms with "will power" alone, the dieter succumbs to the symptom if the hunger or craving becomes too great.

However, when you start the keto diet, eat breakfast which may consist of two eggs and two to three pieces of bacon and one-half to a full avocado. These foods are Keto friendly. They contain four net carbs. Your body doesn't feel deprived of carbs, but four net carbs are a lot less than if you added toast or an English muffin or a biscuit which contains another 22 to 40 net carbs. Those extra high carbs make you feel satisfied for about an hour or two then these carbs crash, and your body start the same hunger symptoms again. By restricting carbs from your diet, you force your body to recondition its energy making and storage systems.

When the body is deprived of carbs, the body must find a new fuel source. Therefore, the body starts manufacturing ketones from the liver to process triglycerides stored as fat.

I may sound like my phonograph needle is stuck, repeating the same information over and over. However, the pure repetition of this information helps you make the transition from a smart beginner to a seasoned pro.

Low Carb Diet

Concisely, you consume a low carb diet (less than 20 carbs per day) making your glucose level fall. The lipase enzyme is produced by the pancreas to digest dietary fats and releases stored triglycerides (Oswald, 2018). These fatty acids travel to the liver, and the liver produces ketones to convert the fatty acids into energy, forcing your body to run on ketones instead of glucose.

High Fat Diet

Good fats are different from bad fats as discussed later. When you start the Keto diet, keep your good fat ratio at 70 to 75% of your total calories and grams. This extra good fat helps the liver produce ketones. This production of ketones is the secret weapon behind your body becoming a fat-burning machine. If you consume a ratio of good fat between 40 to 60%, the process will take longer, and your results may be slower. Don't overdo the consumption of good fat. Ingesting an 80% ratio of good fat does not speed up the fat-burning process.

If you are an athlete and if you consume meat, increase your protein to 30% and adjust the good fat to 60%. Monitor your progress, and adjust your diet from your desired results and your current body condition.

Ketosis

As previously mentioned, ketosis is a metabolic state when the body starts producing an enzyme known as a ketone. The body produces ketones to divide stored fats to produce energy (Mawer, 2018).

Before starting the Keto diet, the body uses glucose to produce energy. Glucose is very easy for the body to produce by dividing simple sugars. However, the bad part of glucose is that the body must use insulin to break down simple sugars. Therefore, it causes the body to have sugar spikes and cravings. When the body ingests too much glucose and can't store it all, it produces the abundance of glucose into triglycerides (Paoli, Bosco, Camporesi, Mangar, 2015).

Understanding how the body interacts with the food groups, you learn how to manipulate your diet and learn how the body enters the state of ketosis. By reducing the intake of carbohydrates, you force the body to produce ketones and start burning fat as fuel.

Ketone Zone

When you first start your Keto diet, you must burn the excess carbohydrates either through your daily routine or through exercise. If you go about your daily routine, it may take a week or two depending on how many carbs were in your carb storage tank. It took me 7 to 10 days to get into ketosis.

If you measure your ketones by either blood stick, urine analysis, or breath analyzer, the ketone level may show 0 to 0.5 millimoles (mM) blood ketones (Musa-Veloso, Likhodii, Cunnane, 2002).

Blood ketones are measured in millimoles (mM). Millimoles per liter (mmol/L) are as follows: a mole is the quantity of a substance containing a number six followed by 23 zeros of atoms (written scientifically as 6.02 x 1023 (Moles, 2019).

A millimole is one-thousandth of a mole. A liter measures fluid volume, which is a little larger than a quart. See chapter on Cooking Conversions for more information on measurements.

This part of the zone is considered pre-ketosis. You may feel hungry between meals, and you may get food cravings if you try fasting for an extended period of time.

I suggest that if you feel hungry or get food cravings to enjoy a low-carb vegetable snack such as a plain celery stick, a cherry tomato, and a green or black olive, or make the Peanut Butter & Chocolate Fat Bomb (see recipes). This snack is easy to make and a great pick-me-up if you're feeling hungry.

If you are experiencing diabetic low sugar symptoms such as shaking or feeling faint, eat something to raise your blood sugar slightly and to curb the symptoms then **consult your medical doctor immediately**.

Crossing the Ketosis Barrier

Crossing the Ketosis Barrier as I call it is when your ketosis level registers between 0.5 and 0.6 mM also known as the Keto flu (Paoli, Bosco, Camporesi, Mangar, 2015; Mawer, 2018). I explain how to stop or cure the symptoms of this barrier in Curing the Keto Flu. If you are crossing this barrier or if you get stuck in this barrier, you may experience fatigue and headaches. Why these symptoms?

Your body is adjusting from burning glucose as an energy source to creating and burning ketones as a fuel source. Your body is also having glucose withdraw symptoms. Don't become alarmed. Your body will adjust, and you and your body will be happier for making it through this transition.

Once you cross this barrier, the symptoms go away, and your body becomes a fat burning machine. Your energy level will go through the roof.

To help your body adjust quicker or easier, bump up your electrolyte level with added salt to your food, drink a cup of bone broth, or take a dietary Keto supplement as explained later in Keto Supplements. I use the Himalayan Pink or Kosher Sea Salt.

Nutritional Ketosis

From 0.61 to 1.0 mM, nutritional ketosis begins. This part of ketosis is the first step toward optimal ketosis. To get to nutritional ketosis, the dieter must restrict carbs below 30 grams per day. Smart beginners and seasoned pros may restrict carbs below 20 grams per day. This phase is called "nutritional" because you are still eating fats and protein; therefore, you are not depriving your body of all nutrients, just carbohydrates.

During this time, you no longer experience food cravings, the Keto flu, and fasting between meals become easier because you are no longer hungry. Most dieters strive to get to nutritional ketosis and usually stop the ketosis process by staying in this zone. In this zone, your body becomes a fat-burning machine.

Keep in mind that dieting is not an exact science. It may take you 4 to 10 days to achieve nutritional ketosis. It took me 7 to 10 days to reach nutritional ketosis. I'm a couch potato at heart, and I lead a sedentary lifestyle most of the time.

Optimal Ketosis

At 1.25 to 2.75 mM, you are in the optimal ketone zone. This part of ketosis is the sweet spot of Keto. To reach this phase, the dieter must restrict carbs to under 20 grams daily. During this phase, the dieter restricts carbs to less than 15 grams daily and calories to less than 800 on specific days then eats regular calories (keeping carbs under 20 grams and calories to 1600 or less) one or two days a week. You pick the days. I discuss this further later in Getting Started and Fasting.

Even though your body becomes a fat-burning machine in nutritional ketosis, this zone turns your body into a well-oiled, fat-burning machine and allows your body to burn fat most efficiently. You gain a huge burst of energy that is truly amazing. If you are a diabetic, you may see that your mg/dl numbers return to or become normal. At this level, I felt like I was 30 years old again.

If you are an athlete, stay in this zone if at all possible. As an athlete, adjust your carb intake to maintain this optimal ketone zone without pushing yourself out of ketosis or into post-exercise or starvation ketosis. I explain this phenomenon further in Getting Kicked Out of Ketosis.

Post Exercise Ketosis

At 2.5 to 3.0 mM, you are entering the post exercise ketosis. This zone is beyond the optimal ketosis, and you may experience diminishing results. The body is still making ketones and burning fat but not as efficient as before. I never experienced this zone.

Starvation Ketosis

From 3.0 to 5.0 mM, you enter starvation ketosis. This part of ketosis is beyond optimal ketosis. To reach this phase, the dieter must restrict all three food groups by fasting. From our cave dwelling days, the human body can fast a few days before starving to death.

In fact, the body can survive without any food for 30 to 40 days so long the dieter stays properly hydrated. Death from starvation occurs from 45 to 61 days, without food and water (Janiszewski, 2015).

Fasting for 24 hours will not put you into starvation ketosis. Even if you tried fasting for 48 to 72 hours straight, you may not achieve starvation ketosis unless you failed to hydrate properly. I expound on fasting and the fasting rules in a later chapter.

Seasoned pros may fast up to 24 hours to shock their systems off diet plateaus; otherwise, I recommend smart beginners stay in nutritional or optimal ketosis, to attain the best weight loss results.

In this part of the zone, you may feel hungry, but the hunger feeling is different than when your body was burning glucose. However, during starvation ketosis, your body is not making ketones or burning fat as efficiently as when you were in nutritional or optimal ketosis. You could experience a prolonged diet plateau period.

I explain how to shock your body off diet plateaus later. This part of the zone is not where you want to be or stay.

Ketoacidosis

From 5.0 to 10 mM, you are entering a dangerous area of ketosis. At 10.0 mM and beyond, you are in ketoacidosis.

For dieters, this ketosis zone is very hard to attain unless you have a medical condition causing your body to produce higher levels of certain hormones such as adrenaline or cortisol (Villines, 2019). This production of these hormones may counter the effect of insulin, triggering diabetic ketoacidosis.

Generally, ketoacidosis is a condition that people with type 1 diabetes experience, which has nothing to do with the Keto diet.

During ketoacidosis, the body experiences brain damage, liver damage, heart damage, kidney failure, or death. Ketoacidosis is a very serious condition.

If you experience ketoacidosis, contact your medical doctor or emergency care provider immediately.

It is very unlikely the diet would cause this situation. However, if your ketone level approaches 4.0 mM or higher, monitor your ketone level closely through testing your ketone level and contact your doctor.

Getting Kicked Out of Ketosis

From time to time, we all get kicked out of ketosis by eating more than 50 grams of carbs in a run of a day or eating or drinking a sugary treat or drink and so on.

At the beginning of your Keto diet, smart beginners need to be careful because your body will wait for an influx of carbs to kick you out of ketosis. Or worse, your body will kick you into the ketosis barrier or even trap you in the barrier for an extended period.

However, when your body gets accustomed to making ketones from your liver, it may take a few more grams of carbs to get kicked out of ketosis (Mawer, 2018; Holland, 2019). Now, your body is accustomed to making ketones and will not switch over because you ate a donut or drank soda.

Your goal, however, should not be how much can you stretch the limit on eating carbs, to see if your body is going to kick you out of ketosis, but to prevent from being kicked out by following a reasonable diet regimen.

If you get kicked out of ketosis, you may experience the fatigue and/or the headaches because you are crossing the ketosis barrier again. Or, it may plop you down in the middle of the ketosis barrier. Either way, you may feel the Keto Flu for a day or so (Hendon, 2020).

To get back into ketosis, you either need to fast, eat low carb meals, drink bone broth, or take a dietary supplement such as BHB.

If you take Keto supplements like the BHB exogenesis supplement, it may help get you back into ketosis. I discuss these dietary supplements further in Keto Supplements.

Continue to track your food even if you are above your carb limit. Never give up. Sometimes by consuming more carbs, this consumption is what your body needs to shock it off a plateau.

Remember, you start each day new and fresh. Forget about the previous day if it wasn't successful.

Keto Testing

To know whether you are in ketosis, you may test your blood ketones with a finger stick similar to diabetes testing, a swab of saliva or breathalyzer testing for Keto, or through urine testing (Musa-Veloso, Likhodii, Cunnane, 2002). Your neighborhood pharmacy may have the supplies for Keto testing, or you can always order the supplies online.

STEP 2
PLAN FOR SUCCESS

Understanding the Food Groups

    Carbohydrates

    Good Carbs

    Bad Carbs

    Net Carbs

    Triglycerides

    Fats

    Good Fats

    Bad Fats

    Proteins

    Fiber

Reading Nutrition Labels

What Foods to Eat

What Foods to Minimize

What Foods to Avoid

What Foods to Stock

Understanding the Food Groups

We rely on these three main food groups and fiber to live. From the day we were hunters and gatherers to our present day, our bodies interact with carbohydrates, fats, and proteins. Fiber provides a balance for carbohydrates, fats, and proteins.

In this chapter, I examine what these food groups are and how these groups interact with the body. I empower you with the advantages and disadvantages of the food groups, how to read nutrition labels, what foods to eat, what foods to minimize, what foods to avoid, and what foods to stock in your pantry. I explain the Keto supplements and apple cider vinegar.

Understanding how these food groups work with your body, you are now empowered to proceed on your weight loss journey.

Carbohydrates

Carbohydrates or carbs can also be defined chemically as neutral compounds of carbon, hydrogen and oxygen (Shiel, Jr., 2018).

Three types of carbs exist: sugars, starches and fiber. Simple carbohydrates, or sugars, occur naturally in foods such as fruit (fructose) and milk (lactose) or come from refined sources such as table sugar (sucrose) or corn syrup. The rule of thumb is if the suffix contains **-ose**, don't consume it. These types of carbs are bad.

The body breaks down most sugars and starches into glucose, a simple sugar that the body uses to feed cells. In fact, the body loves to break down simple sugars and carbs because the body doesn't have to work very hard to convert these elements into glucose.

Almost every food item contains carbs, but not all carbs are created equal. Carbs from leafy vegetables are different than carbs from pasta, rice, bread, or sugar (Shiel, Jr., 2018).

Most people consume from 200 to 500 grams or about 45 to 65 percent of carbs in 2000 calories per day, and unfortunately some consume well over a 1000 grams of carbs per day. The Standard Keto Diet (SKD) restricts that percentage to 5% or about 20 grams for strict Keto and 50 grams for the not-so-strict Keto. That's a huge difference for a dieter to get accustomed to in a short period. Dieters can adapt to this change if they proceed slowly. Start with consuming 2000 calories and about 50 grams of carbs for the first few days to a week. Then adjust your diet plan to subtract unnecessary calories and carbs until you are consuming less than 1200 calories and 20 grams of carbs per day. If you aren't getting the results you want, adjust your diet plan until you find your happy medium (Gunnars, 2018).

Remember, diets are not an exact science. Everyone's body is different. To find what works for you, don't be afraid to adjust the intake of carbs, fats, and proteins until you find what works for you.

When the body runs low on glucose, it craves more carbs.

The body processes and adsorbs carbs found in bread, rice, pasta, sweets, processed food, and simple sugars a lot faster than the carbs found in vegetables. The rule of thumb is that the tougher the time the body has to process and break down macronutrients, the less likely it adsorbs the nutrient. This means if the body has a hard time breaking down some food items or nutrients, most likely the body will discard those items such as fiber during the waste process. A generation or two ago, farmers could consume sugar cane off the stalk.

The body had a tough time processing raw sugar cane; therefore, the body sent most of the sugar or sugar cane to waste.

Carbs are the sugars, starches and fibers found in fruits, grains, vegetables and milk products.

Advantages

The following list shows the advantages of carbs:

- Provides energy

- Regulates blood glucose

- Prevents bone loss and degradation of other tissues

- Keep proteins from being broken down for energy

Disadvantages

- The following list shows the disadvantages of carbs:

- Allows weight gain

- Increases risk for Type 2 Diabetes, heart disease, and other health disorders

- Creates brain fog

- Elevates blood pressure, cholesterol, and triglyceride levels

- Thickens arteries

DO NOT EAT BAD CARBS

Fruit:

Apples

Bananas

Citrus fruits

Kiwifruit

Melons

Legumes:

Beans

Chickpeas

Lentils

Soybeans

Milk products:

Milk

Soy

Tofu

Processed Foods:

Candy

Corn meal

Flour (bread, pasta, cakes, other pastries)

Pre-packaged or prepared foods

Sodas

Sugar

Sugary drinks

Starchy vegetables:

Carrots

Corn

Peas

Potatoes

Sweet potatoes

Yams

Whole grain foods:

Amaranth

Barley

Bread

Breakfast cereals

Oatmeal

Pasta

Quinoa

Rice

Good Carbs

Good carbs are found in leafy vegetables. Fiber is also a carb. It could be considered a good carb. Smart beginners still cannot overeat these carbs, though no one has ever overeaten vegetable-based carbs, that I know of, because your body lets you know right away when it has had enough vegetables. The best part of these carbs is the body has a tougher time breaking them down into glucose.

DO EAT GOOD CARBS

Fruit (eat in moderation, no more than 2 to 6 berries each):

Blackberries

Blueberries

Raspberries

Strawberries

Non-starchy vegetables:

Asparagus

Broccoli

Cabbage

Cauliflower

Cucumber

Green beans

Leafy greens

Mushrooms

Peppers

Tomatoes

Zucchini

Nuts and seeds (eat in moderation, no more than 15 nuts total):

Almonds

Cashews

Peanuts

Pistachios

Pumpkin seeds

Sunflower seeds

Walnuts

Milk Products:

Almond milk

Cashew milk

Soy milk

Bad Carbs

The bad carbs are the ones the body has no trouble processing such as sugar, simple sugars, and processed food. The body loves these carbs because it doesn't have to work hard to process these foods. However, if you continue to eat these bad carbs, you can develop health issues such as heart disease, diabetes, obesity, and so on. Refer to the food list on What Foods to Avoid.

Net Carbs

When shopping, calculate the net carbs on the nutrition labels. Food companies are not going to put this information readily available to you because all processed food is bad for you. They want you to stay uninformed.

I provide the following equation showing Net Carbs equal Carbohydrates minus Fiber, written as:

Carbs – Fiber = Net Carbs

Triglycerides

Think. If the body's carb storage is like a gas tank, a smaller connecting sub tank is the triglycerides tank used as an overflow tank. The smaller tank receives the overflow of glucose from carbs called triglycerides.

When the body fills up on carbs where the carb tank is full or overflowing, the excess carbs becomes triglycerides. When the triglyceride tank becomes full or nearly full, the body empties it and stores the triglycerides as belly fat. The body is resourceful by storing it as belly fat or other fat on the arms, legs, shoulders, back or wherever the body has room.

Even worse, the body may convert this fat into its more dangerous cousin called "visceral fat" and store it around vital organs such as the heart, liver, stomach, intestines, and so on.

The body always accommodates these fat cells and finds room for them. The body never hangs out a NO VACANCY SIGN for any kinds of fat especially visceral fat (Gotter, 2017).

If you are diabetic and if your carbs are running away with your health, your triglycerides are also a nemesis to your health.

To lower your blood sugar and your triglyceride level, you limit your carb intake to 5% or less than 20 g per day. After about two weeks and if you test your blood glucose, you should notice that your numbers are either normal or returning to normal.

It also helps if you exercise at least one or two days a week. I expound on exercise in a later chapter.

On Keto, by eating a low carb diet, you can quickly empty your carb and triglyceride tank. As I previously stated, it took me 7 to 10 days before I entered the state of ketosis. My glucose readings ran away at over 200 mg/dl daily then dropped to 75 to 90 mg/dl daily when I started Keto. According to the medical websites, any glucose reading under 100 mg/dl is considered normal (WebMD, 2018).

Fats

Fats are any of numerous compounds of carbon, hydrogen, and oxygen that make up most of animal or plant fat and are important to nutrition as sources of energy. Fat gets a bad rap. For over 50 years, medical scientist, practitioners, dieticians, and so on claimed that fats are bad and leads to heart disease and death. Good fats, like the poor egg, fall in and out of favor with this group.

Throughout my lifetime, the medical influencers announced that the egg is good for you, and then a few years later they say the egg is bad for you. A few years later, the egg is good again. I know medicine is not an exact science but come on. Either the egg is good or bad. And, fats are good or bad.

Good Fats

Good fats are monounsaturated and polyunsaturated fats. **These fats do not make you fat.** However, be aware good fat foods contain a powerful punch in the number of calories, and don't eat more than the recommended serving per meal.

Nutritionally speaking, monounsaturated fatty acids are fatty acids with one double bond in the fatty acid chain with the remainder carbon atoms being single bonded. Polyunsaturated fatty acids contain more than one double bond. Who cares about that? What are the good fats and what are the benefits?

DO EAT THESE FOODS CONTAINING GOOD FATS

Monounsaturated fat foods:

Avocados

Nuts: Almonds, Brazil Nuts, Cashews, Macadamia Nuts, Peanuts, Pistachios

Olives

Olive oil (Extra Virgin Olive Oil)

Peanut butter (with < 5 net carbs)

Polyunsaturated fat foods:

Fish: Albacore tuna, Herring, Mackerel, Salmon, Trout

Flax seeds or flax oil

Sunflower seeds

Walnuts

The following list shows the benefits from these foods:

- Promotes heart health

- Decreases the risk of heart disease and stroke

- Lowers LDL (bad) cholesterol

- Increases HDL (good) cholesterol

- Supports cell growth

- Protects organs

- Keeps the body warm

- Helps the body absorb some nutrients

- Produces important hormones

- Promotes normal brain functions and nervous system

- Protects against dry eye disease

- Reduces inflammation

- Gives you energy

Bad Fats

Bad fats are unimportant fats you can eliminate from your diet. These bad fats are as follows:

- Saturated fats: these fats are different from monounsaturated and polyunsaturated fats

- Trans fats: fats result from the hydrogenation process, which occurs when hydrogen is added.

Foods containing trans fats:

- Fast food

- Fried food

- Shortening

- Processed and prepackaged food

Advantages

- None

Disadvantages

- Raises LDL (bad) cholesterol

- Increases the risk for heart disease and stroke.

The rule of thumb is if man has created, handled, or augmented these fats, smart beginners know not to eat these fats.

Proteins

Proteins are any class of nitrogenous organic compounds containing amino acids, compounds and carbon, hydrogen, oxygen, nitrogen and sometimes sulfur. Proteins are a type of nutrient found in meats such as **beef, pork, poultry,** and **fish**. See the meat section of What Foods to Eat for further details.

Advantages

- Reduces appetite cravings and binge eating

- Lowers hunger levels

- Increases muscle mass and strength

- Provides nutrients for bones

- Boosts metabolism and increases fat burning

- Promotes weight loss causing the dieter to eat less calories

- Provides sustained energy

- Promotes better skin, hair, and nails

- Allows better workout exercising

- Permits better sleep

- Builds, repairs, and maintains tissue

- Boost the immune system

- Lowers blood glucose

Disadvantages

- Makes weight loss temporary unless dieter continues to diet

- Stores excess consumed proteins as fat and the surplus of amino acids are excreted

- Contains higher calories than some non-protein foods

- Ensures weight gain if proteins are overeaten

- Increases cancer risk

- Bad breath

- Constipation or diarrhea

- Dehydration

- Kidney damage

- Heart disease

Even though these disadvantages seem daunting, dieters should look at the positive outcome that protein offers with weight loss than concentrating on the disadvantages.

Fiber

Fiber is carbohydrates the body CANNOT digest. These carbs pass through the body and is discarded as waste. The good part about fiber is that it sometime attaches to other carbs or it blocks other carbs from being absorbed by the body. Therefore, fiber is truly the good carb.

Dietary fiber or roughage is the portion of plant-derived food, which cannot be completely broken down by human digestive enzymes.

Advantages

- Reduces the risk of chronic diseases

- Promotes normal bowel movements and helps maintain bowel or gut health

- Lowers cholesterol levels

- Helps control blood sugar levels

- Slows the rate that sugar is absorbed into the blood stream

- Attaches to other carbs and helps the body eliminate them

- Passes through the body undigested

- Aids in weight loss and helps achieve healthy weight

- Flushes cholesterol and harmful carcinogens from the body

DO EAT THESE FOODS FOR FIBER

- Chia seeds

- Dark Leafy Vegetables

- Nuts

- Popcorn

- Raspberries

- Strawberries

My best recommendation on food with fiber is to study the nutrition label to see if the food contains plenty of fiber. I hunt for foods containing 5 grams of fiber or more. These foods literally are the fiber gold mines.

DO NOT EAT THESE FOODS FOR FIBER

- Juices

- Grains or refined grains

- Oats

Like fats, the rule of thumb is if man has created, handled, or augmented these foods touting fiber or high in fiber, the smart beginner does not make these processed foods part of their diet regimen.

Reading Nutrition Labels

Reading nutrition labels for the first time is a daunting task for everyone. In the beginning, I never looked at a nutrition label because I felt unsure on how to read it. Plus, I convinced myself each label read differently on purpose to confuse the average consumer. My suspicions were correct. Food corporations tend to hide facts in clear sight on the label.

Smart beginners must become good detectives to find Keto-friendly foods by reading nutrition labels. This chapter demystifies nutritional labels. By the time you finish reading this chapter, you will be a seasoned pro at reading and understanding nutritional labels.

I created the following nutrition label from my recollection of reading past labels. The information on this label pertains to no specific product or item. Any part of this label resembling a real nutrition label is strictly coincidental. This label is for demonstration purposes only.

Nutrition Facts	
Serving Size 1 piece (30 g) Serving Per Container about 6	
Amount Per Serving	
Calories 240	Calories from Fat 50
	% Daily Value
Total Fat 6 g	9%
Saturated Fat 0.5 g	3%
Trans Fat 0 g	
Cholesterol 5 mg	2%
Sodium 390	20%
Total Carbohydrates 10 g	10%
Dietary Fiber 4 g	12%
Sugars 2 g	
Protein 6 g	
Vitamin A 4%	Vitamin C 8%
Calcium 0%	Iron 10%

I summarized Dr. Kennedy's article (n.d.) *Learning to read labels* so that smart beginners may read nutrition labels effectively with the following steps:

1.   Look for the serving size and serving per container.

Nutrition Facts	
Serving Size 1 piece (30 g) Serving Per Container about 6	
Amount Per Serving	
Calories 240	Calories from Fat 50
	% Daily Value

2.   Compare the portion size to the serving size.

On the label above, the serving size is 1 piece or 30 grams if measured by weight.

The number of servings per container is about 6. This product is a solid. If you ate the entire package contents, the nutritional facts on this label would be multiplied by six.

3.   Find the total calorie count and total calories per serving.

On this part of the label, if you ate the entire package contents, you'd consumed about 1440 total calories with 300 calories from Fat.

Nutrition Facts	
Serving Size 1 piece (30 g) Serving Per Container about 6	
Amount Per Serving	
Calories 240	Calories from Fat 50
	% Daily Value

Don't concern yourself with the daily values found on the right side. These values pertain to the number of grams found in Fat, Cholesterol, Sodium, Carbohydrates, Fiber, Sugar, and Protein from the number of daily requirements as prescribed or suggested by the government. The government requires food companies to compare the quantity of the above listed macronutrients to the daily 2,000-calorie diet requirement.

4. Look for the Total Carbohydrates minus the Dietary Fiber.

From the example label, this item has 10 grams total carbs minus 4 grams of fiber. Therefore, this label shows that this item has 6 grams of net carbs.

Trans Fat 0 g	
Cholesterol 5 mg	2%
Sodium 390	20%
Total Carbohydrates 10 g	10%
Dietary Fiber 4 g	12%
Sugars 2 g	
Protein 6 g	

If you track other macronutrients such as Fats, Sodium, Cholesterol, Sugar, and Protein, the number of these items are listed in grams also.

What Foods to Eat

The following list is alphabetized for easy read and convenience. This list contains the serving size, calories (kcal), fat, carbs, fiber, and protein. This list is for those who are following any of the Keto diets. Also note the items contain less than 7 grams of net carbs per serving.

The nutritional facts are estimated and provided as a courtesy. The nutritional facts are generated by an online API which recognizes ingredient names and amounts and makes calculations from the serving size with algorithms. Results may vary.

Sources: nutritionix.com, carb manager app, or fatsecret.com.

Cheeses

Blue, 1 cup crumbled (135 g): 477 kcal | fat 39 g | carbs 3.2 g | fiber 0 g | protein 29 g

Brie, 1 cup, sliced (144 g): 480 kcal | fat 40 g | carbs 0.6 g | fiber 0 g | protein 30 g

Cheddar, 1 slice (1 ounce or 28 g): 113 kcal | fat 9 g | carbs 0.4 g | fiber 0 g | protein 7 g

Colby, 1 slice (1 ounce or 28 g): 110 kcal | fat 9 g | carbs 0.7 g | fiber 0 g | protein 7 g

Cottage Cheese, ½ cup, small curd (not packed) (112.5 g): 111 kcal | fat 5 g | carbs 4 g | fiber 0 g | protein 12.5 g

Cream Cheese, 1 package, small (3 ounce or 85 g): 291 kcal | fat 29 g | carbs 3.5 g | fiber 0 g | protein 5 g

Feta, 1 cup, crumbled (150 g) is 396 kcal | total fat 32 g | carbs 6 g | fiber 0 g | protein 21 g

Goat Cheese, 1 ounce (28.4 g) is 103 kcal | total fat 8 g | carbs 0 g | fiber 0 g | protein 6 g

Gouda, 1 ounce (28.4 g) is 101 kcal | total fat 8 g | carbs 0.6 g | fiber 0 g | protein 7 g

Gruyere, 1 slice (1 ounce or 28 g) is 116 kcal | total fat 9 g | carbs 0.1 g | fiber 0 g | protein 8 g

Monterey Jack, 1 cup, shredded (113 g) is 422 kcal | total fat 34 g | net carbs 0.8 g | fiber 0 g | protein 30 g

Mozzarella, 1 slice (1 ounce or 28 g) is 78 kcal | total fat 4.8 g | carbs 0.9 g | fiber 0 g | protein 8 g

Parmesan or **Parmigiano-Reggiano**, 1 tablespoon (5 g) is 22 kcal | total fat 1.4 g | carbs 0.2 g | fiber 0 g | protein 1.9 g

Ricotta, 1 cup (246 g) is 428 kcal | total fat 32 g | carbs 7 g | fiber 0 g | protein 28 g

String Cheese, 1 piece (28 g) is 80 kcal | total fat 6 g | carbs 1 g | fiber 0 g | protein 6 g

Swiss, 1 slice (1 ounce or 28 g) is 106 kcal | total fat 8 g | carbs 1.5 g | fiber 0 g | protein 8 g

Cooking / Baking – Fats & Oils

Bacon Fat, 1 teaspoon (4.3 g) is 39 kcal | total fat 4.3 g | carbs 0 g | fiber 0 g | protein 0 g

Béarnaise Sauce, 2 tablespoons (32 g) is 155 kcal | total fat 17 g | carbs 0.7 g | fiber 0.1 g | protein 0.9 g

Butter, 1 tablespoon (14 g) is 102 kcal | total fat 12 g | carbs 0 g | fiber 0 g | protein 0.1 g

Coconut Oil, 1 tablespoon (13.6 g) is 117 kcal | total fat 14 g | carbs 0 g | fiber 0 g | protein 0 g

Hollandaise Sauce, 1 ounce (28.3 g) is 78 kcal | total fat 6.9 g | carbs 3.1 g | fiber 0 g | protein 0.6 g

Olive Oil (Extra Virgin Olive Oil), 1 tablespoon (13.5 g) is 119 kcal | total fat 14 g | carbs 0 g | fiber 0 g | protein 0 g

Peanut Oil, 1 tablespoon (13.5 g) is 119 kcal | total fat 14 g | carbs 0 g | fiber 0 g | protein 0 g

Sesame Oil, 1 tablespoon (13.6 g) is 120 kcal | total fat 14 g | carbs 0 g | fiber 0 g | protein 0 g

Sunflower Oil, 1 tablespoon (13.6 g) is 120 kcal | total fat 14 g | carbs 0 g | fiber 0 g | protein 0 g

Cooking / Baking – Flour, Powder & Seeds

Almond Flour, ¼ cup (56.7 g) is 150 kcal; total fat 11 g | carbs 6 g | fiber 3 g | protein 6 g

Almond Flakes, 4-½ teaspoons (25 g) are 161 kcal | total fat 14 g | carbs 1.6 g | fiber 1.9 g | protein 6.4 g

Chia Seeds, 1 ounce (28.4 g) is 138 kcal | total fat 9 g | carbs 12 g | fiber 10 g | protein 4.7 g

Cocoa Powder (Over 70% Cacao), 1 tablespoon (5 g) is 21 kcal | total fat 0.5 g | carbs 3 g | fiber 1 g | protein 1.1 g

Coconut Flour, 2 tablespoons (14 g) are 60 kcal | total fat 1.5 g | carbs 9 g | fiber 5 g | protein 3 g

Coconut Flakes, ¼ cup (15 g) is 100 kcal | total fat 8 g | carbs 5 g | fiber 3 g | protein 1 g

Flax Meal, 2 tablespoons (13 g) are 70 kcal | total fat 4.5 g | carbs 4 g | fiber 3 g | protein 3 g

Flax Seeds, 1-½ tablespoon (10 g) is 53 kcal | total fat 4 g | carbs 3 g | fiber 3 g | protein 2.5 g

Dairy

Greek Yogurt, 1 container (170 g) is 100 kcal | total fat 0.7 g | carbs 6 g | fiber 0 g | protein 17 g

Heavy Whipping Cream, 1 tablespoon (15 g) is 29 kcal | total fat 2.9 g | carbs 0.5 g | fiber 0 g | protein 0.4 g

Mayonnaise, 1 tablespoon (13.8 g) is 94 kcal | total fat 10 g | carbs 0.1 g | fiber 0 g | protein 0.1 g

Sour Cream, 1 tablespoon (12 g) is 23 kcal | total fat 2.4 g | carbs 0.3 g | fiber 0 g | protein 0.2 g

Fruits

Apricot, 1 each (35 g) is 17 kcal | total fat 0.1 g | carbs 3.9 g | fiber 0.7 g | protein 0.5 g

Avocado, 1 small (100 g) is 160 kcal | total fat 15 g | carbs 9 g | fiber 7 g | protein 2 g

Blackberry, 10 berries (51 g) are 21.9 kcal | total fat 0.3 g | carbs 4.9 g | fiber 2.7 g | protein 0.7 g

Blueberry, 10 berries are 7.8 kcal | total fat 0.0 g | carbs 2.0 g | fiber 0.3 g | protein 0.1 g

Cherries, 1 cherry is 5.2 kcal | total fat 0.0 g | carbs 1.3 g | fiber 0.2 | protein 0.7 g

Cranberries, ½ cup (1.8 ounces or 50 g) is 23 kcal | total fat 0.1 g | carbs 6 g | fiber 1.8 g | protein 0 g

Lemon, 1 fruit (2-⅛ inch diameter) (58 g) is 16.8 kcal | total fat 0.2 g | carbs 5.4 g | fiber 1.6 g | protein 0.6 g

Lime, 1 fruit, 2-inch diameter (67 g) is 20 kcal | total fat 0.1 g | carbs 7.1 g | fiber 1.9 g | protein 0.5 g

Passion Fruit, 1 fruit without refuse (18 g) is 17.5 kcal | total fat 0.1 g | carbs 4.2 g | fiber 1.9 | protein 0.4 g

Raspberries, 10 berries (19 g) are 10 kcal | total fat 0.1 g | carbs 2.3 g | fiber 1.2 g | protein 0.2 g

Rhubarb, 1 cup, diced (122 g) is 25.6 kcal | total fat 0.2 g | carbs 5.5 g | fiber 2.2 g | protein 1.1 g

Strawberries, 1 medium (1-¼ inch diameter) (12 g) is 3.8 kcal | total fat 0 g | carbs 0.9 g | fiber 0.2 g | protein 0.1 g

Tomato, Grape, 1 each (0.3 ounces or 8 g) is 1.4 kcal | total fat 0 g | carbs 0.3 g | fiber 0.1 g | protein 0.1 g

Liquids

Almond Milk, Unsweetened, 1 cup (8.5 ounces or 240 ml) is 30.4 kcal | total fat 2.5 g | carbs 1.1 g | fiber 0.6 g | protein 1 g

Bulletproof Coffee, (see recipe) 1 tall cup (16 fluid ounces or 474 g) is 1197 kcal | total fat 132 g | carbs 2.7 g | fiber 0 g | protein 2.7 g

Cashew Milk, Unsweetened, 1 cup (8.5 ounces or 240 ml) is 25 kcal | total fat 2 g | carbs 1 g | fiber 0 g | protein 1.0 g

Coconut Milk, 1 tablespoon (1.1 ounces or 30 g) is 60.6 kcal | total fat 6.2 g | carbs 1.7 g | fiber 0.3 g | protein 0.5 g

Coffee (Black), 1 tall cup (16 fluid ounces or 474 g) is 4.7 kcal | total fat 0.1 g | carbs 2.2 g | fiber 2.2 g | protein 0.6 g

Green Tea, Brewed, Unsweetened, 8 fluid ounces (237 g) is 2.4 kcal | total fat 0 g | carbs 0 g | fiber 0 g | protein 0.5 g

Soymilk, 1 cup (243 g) is 100 kcal | total fat 4 g | carbs 8 g | fiber 1 g | protein 7 g

Meat – Beef

Don't shy away from well marbled meats with fat by buying lean cuts of meat. The body needs the good fat that reduces from the meat, and the fat gives the meat flavor.

Beef Bone Broth, one 8 fluid ounce cup (240 ml) is 48 kcal | total fat 0.3 g | carbs 0.7 g | fiber 0 g | protein 10 g

Beef Short Ribs, 3 ounces (85 g) are 302 kcal | total fat 24.2 g | carbs 0 g | fiber (not given) | protein 19.6 g

Corned Beef, 3 ounces (85 g) are 213 kcal | total fat 16 g | carbs 0.4 g | fiber 0 g | protein 15 g

Hamburger, Ground, 1 pound (453.6 g) is 1506 kcal | total fat 136 g | carbs 0 g | fiber 0 g | protein 65 g

Prime Rib, 8 ounces of boneless are 603 kcal | total fat 39.28 g | carbs 0 g | fiber 0 g | protein 58.77 g

Roast Beef, 1 thin slice (approx. 4-½" x 2-½" x ⅛") is 56 kcal | total fat 3.64 g | carbs 0 g | fiber 0 g | protein 5.44 g

Steak, Ribeye, 4 ounces (112 g) are 280 kcal | total fat 20 g | carbs 0 g | fiber 0 g | protein 22 g

Steak, T-Bone, (Trimmed to ¼" Fat), 6 ounces are 361 kcal | total fat 24.34 g | carbs 0 g | fiber 0 g | protein 32.98 g

Steak, Top Sirloin, (Trimmed to ⅛" Fat), 5 ounces are 285 kcal | total fat 18.02 g | carbs 0 g | fiber 0 g | protein 28.78 g

Meat – Chicken

Chicken Bone Broth, Organic, 1 cup (8 ounces) is 45 kcal | total fat 0.5 g | carbs 1 g | fiber 0 g | protein 9 g

Cornish Hen, 1 roasted hen (1-¼ pound, raw) (yield after cooking, bone removed) is 793 kcal | total fat 55.48 g | carbs 0 g | fiber 0 g | protein 67.87 g

Egg, Boiled, 1 large is 77 kcal | total fat 5.28 g | carbs 0.56 g | fiber 0 g | protein 6.26 g

Egg, fried (over-hard), 1 large is 92 kcal | total fat 7.04 g | carbs 0.4 g | fiber 0 g | protein 6.27 g

Egg, Scrambled, 1 large eggs are 101 kcal | total fat 7.45 g | carbs 1.34 g | fiber 0 g | protein 6.76 g

Egg, Raw, 1 large is 74 kcal | total fat 4.97 g | carbs 0.38 g | fiber 0 g | protein 6.29 g

Ground Chicken, 1 cup (cooked) is 301 kcal | total fat 17.13 g | carbs 0 g | fiber 0 g | protein 34.38 g

Legs, 1 small (yield after cooking, bone removed) (skin eaten) is 212 kcal | total fat 12.28 g | carbs 0 g | fiber 0 g | protein 23.68 g

Tenders, Breast (Perdue), 1 piece (35.5 g) are 80 kcal | total fat 3.5 g | carbs 6 g | fiber 0 g | protein 5 g

Thigh, 1 small (yield after cooking, bone removed) is 135 kcal | total fat 8.45 g | carbs 0 g | fiber 0 g | protein 13.67 g

Whole Rotisserie Chicken, 1 serving, 3 ounces are 170 kcal | total fat 10 g | carbs 0 g | fiber 0 g | protein 18 g

Wing, 1 small (yield after cooking, bone removed) is 81 kcal | total fat 5.4 g | carbs 0 g | fiber 0 g | protein 7.46 g

Meat – Other Poultry

Duck Egg, Raw, 1 egg is 130 kcal | total fat 9.64 g | carbs 1.02 g | fiber 0 g | protein 8.97 g

Duck, Roasted, 1/2 breast (yield after cooking, bone removed) is 255 kcal | total fat 21.46 g | carbs 0 g | fiber 0 g | protein 14.37 g

Goose Egg, Raw, 1 egg is 266 kcal | total fat 19.11 g | carbs 1.94 g | fiber 0 g | protein 19.97 g

Goose, Roasted Wild, 3 ounces with bone (yield after cooking, bone removed) are 173 kcal | total fat 12.44 g | carbs 0 g | fiber 0 g | protein 14.28 g

Pheasant Eggs, 1 egg is 135 kcal | total fat 9.4 g | carbs 0.9 g | fiber 0 g | protein 11 g

Pheasant, ½ breast (yield after cooking, bone removed) is 312 kcal | total fat 15.3 g | carbs 0 g | fiber 0 g | protein 40.97 g

Quail Egg, Raw, 1 egg is 14 kcal | total fat 1 g | carbs 0.04 g | fiber 0 g | protein 1.17 g

Quail, 1 quail (yield after cooking, bone removed) is 177 kcal | total fat 10.67 g | carbs 0 g | fiber 0 g | protein 19 g

Meat – Pork

Bacon, Applewood Smoked, 2 slices (20 g) is 110 kcal | total fat 9 g | carbs 0 g | fiber 0 g | protein 5 g

Ground Pork 80/20, 4 ounces (112 g) are 280 kcal | total fat 22 g | carbs 1 g | fiber 0 g | protein 19 g

Ham, Fried, 1 thin slice (approx. 4-½" x 2-½" x ⅛") is 47 kcal | total fat 3.15 g | carbs 0.07 g | fiber 0 g | protein 4.32 g

Pork Chops, 1 small or thin cut (3 oz, with bone, raw) (yield after cooking, bone removed) is 118 kcal | total fat 6.85 g | carbs 0 g | fiber 0 g | protein 13.12 g

Pork Roast, 1 thin slice (approx. 4-½" x 2-½" x ⅛") is 52 kcal | total fat 3.06 g | carbs 0 g | fiber 0 g | protein 5.67 g

Meat – Seafood

Albacore Tuna, White in Water, 2 ounces (56 g) are 60 kcal | total fat 1 g | carbs 0 g | fiber 0 g | protein 12 g

Albacore Tuna, Wild Caught, 4 ounces (113 g) are 120 kcal | total fat 1 g | carbs 0 g | fiber 0 g | protein 25 g

Catfish, Fried Battered, 1 fillet (5" x 2-½" x 3/8") is 182 kcal | total fat 12.8 g | carbs 5.03 g | fiber 0.2 g | protein 11.12 g

Herring, 1 ounce boneless is 45 kcal | total fat 2.56 g | carbs 0 g | fiber 0 g | protein 5.09 g

Mackerel, 2-ounce boneless is 95 kcal | total fat 5.31 g | carbs 0 g | fiber 0 g | protein 10.95 g

Mahi Mahi, 1 fillet is 100 kcal | total fat 0.82 g | carbs 0 g | fiber 0 g | protein 21.76 g

Salmon, 4-ounce boneless is 166 kcal | total fat 6.72 g | carbs 0 g | fiber 0 g | protein 24.52 g

Trout, Mixed Species, 1 fillet is 117 kcal | total fat 5.22 g | carbs 0 g | fiber 0 g | protein 16.41 g

Meat – Turkey

Turkey Bacon, 1 thin slice (yield after cooking) is 31 kcal | total fat 2.23 g | carbs 0.25 g | fiber 0 g | protein 2.37 g

Turkey Breast (with skin), 3-ounce boneless is 134 kcal | total fat 5.97 g | carbs 0 g | fiber 0 g | protein 18.62 g

Deli Turkey Meat, 1 slice (1 ounce) is 29 kcal | total fat 0.47 g | carbs 1.19 g | fiber 0.1 g | protein 4.84 g

Ground Turkey (85/15), 4 ounces (112 g) are 220 kcal | total fat 17 g | carbs 0 g | fiber 0 g | protein 19 g

Turkey Drumstick, Roasted, 1 small (from hen, approx. 11- to 13-pound bird) (yield after cooking, bone removed) is 255 kcal | total fat 12.08 g | carbs 0 g | fiber 0 g | protein 34.27 g

Turkey Sausage, 1 ounce is 44 kcal | total fat 2.29 g | carbs 0.13 g | fiber 0 g | protein 5.33 g

Whole Turkey (Butterball), per 4 ounces (112 g) is 160 kcal | total fat 4.5 g | carbs 0 g | fiber 0 g | protein 28 g

Miscellaneous

Tofu, 0.2 block (91 g) is 76 kcal | total fat 4.8 g | carbs 1.1 g | fiber 0.9 g | protein 9.1 g

Nuts & Seeds

Almonds, Raw, 10 almonds are 70 kcal | total fat 6.1 g | carbs 2.4 g | fiber 0.1 g | protein 2.6 g

Brazil Nuts, Raw, ¼ cup or 12 nuts (30 g) are 200 kcal | total fat 20 g carbs 4 g | fiber 2 g | protein 4 g

Cashews, Raw Whole, ⅛ cup (15 g) are 90 kcal | total fat 6.5 g | carbs 4.5 g | fiber 0.5 g | protein 3.5 g

Macadamia Nuts, 1 ounce or 10 to 12 nuts are 204 kcal | total fat 21.48 g | net carbs 3.92 g | fiber 2.4 g | protein 2.24 g

Peanuts, Dry Roasted, Unsalted, 10 nuts are 60 kcal | total fat 5 g | net carbs 2.1 g | protein 2.4 g

Peanuts, In Shell (Shell not eaten), 1 cup edible yield is 305 kcal | total fat 26.78 g | carbs 7.78 g | fiber 4.8 g | protein 14.3 g

Pecans, Chopped, ¼ cup (28 g) is 200 kcal | total fat 20 g | carbs 4 g | fiber 3 g | protein 3 g

Pecans, Halves, ¼ cup (28 g) is 190 kcal | total fat 20 g | carbs 4 g | fiber 3 g | protein 3 g

Pecans, Raw, ¼ cup (30 g) is 210 kcal | total fat 21 g | carbs 4 g | fiber 2 g | protein 3 g

Pistachio Nuts, 1 ounce or 49 kernels are 158 kcal | total fat 12.6 g | carbs 7.93 g | fiber 2.9 g | protein 5.84 g

Pumpkin Seeds, Raw, ¼ cup (30 g) is 170 kcal | total fat 15 g | carbs 3 g | fiber 2 g | protein 9 g

Sunflower Seeds, Raw, ¼ cup (30 g) is 170 kcal | total fat 15 g | carbs 6 g | fiber 3 g | protein 7 g

Sunflower Seeds, In Shell, 1 package (95 g) is 180 kcal | total fat 15 g | carbs 4 g | fiber 3 g | protein 6 g

Walnuts, Organic, ¼ cup (28 g) is 180 kcal | total fat 17 g | carbs 5 g | fiber 1 g | protein 4 g

Sauces/Dressings

Blue Cheese Dressing, Chunky (Kraft), 2 tablespoons (30 g) are 120 kcal | total fat 12 g | carbs 2 g | fiber 0 g | protein 1 g

Italian Salad Dressing (Wishbone), 2 tablespoons (30 ml) are 80 kcal | total fat 7 g | carbs 4 g | fiber 0 g | protein 0 g

Lemon Juice, 100% (Great Value), 1 teaspoon (5 ml) is 0 kcal | total fat 0 g | carbs 0 g | fiber 0 g | protein 0 g

Lime Juice, 100%, 1 teaspoon (5 ml) is 0 kcal | total fat 0 g | carbs 0 g | fiber 0 g | protein 0 g

Mustard, Classic Yellow (French's), 1 teaspoon (5 g) is 0 kcal | total fat 0 g | carbs 0 g | fiber 0 g | protein 0 g

Mustard, Dijon, 1 teaspoon (5 g) is 4 kcal | total fat 0.19 g | carbs 0.47 g | fiber 0.2 g | protein 0.24 g

Mustard, Spicy Brown (Gulden's), 1 teaspoon (5 g) is 5 kcal | total fat 0 g | carbs 0 g | fiber 0 g | protein 0 g

Ranch Dressing Original (Hidden Valley), 2 tablespoons (30 ml) are 140 kcal | total fat 14 g | carbs 2 g | fiber 0 g | protein 0 g

Salsa, Picante Medium (Pace), 2 tablespoons (32 g) are 8 kcal | total fat 0 g | carbs 2 g | fiber 1 g | protein 0 g

Soy Sauce (Kikkoman), 1 tablespoon (0.5 ounce) is 10 kcal | total fat 0 g | carbs 1 g | fiber 0 g | protein 2 g

Vinegar, Apple Cider, 1 tablespoon (14.9 g) is 3 kcal | total fat 0 g | carbs 0.1 g | fiber 0 g | protein 0 g

Vinegar, Balsamic, 1 tablespoon (16 g) is 14 kcal | total fat 0 g | carbs 2.7 g | fiber 0 g | protein 0.1 g

Worcestershire Sauce (Lea & Perrins), 1 tablespoon (15 ml) is 5 kcal | total fat 0 g | net carbs 1 g | protein 0 g

Spices

Bacon Bits (Real Fully Cooked), 1 tablespoon (7 g) is 33 kcal | total fat 1.8 g | carbs 2 g | fiber 0.7 g | protein 2.2 g

Capers drained, 1 tablespoon (8.6 g) is 2 kcal | total fat 0.1 g | carbs 0.4 g | fiber 0.3 g | protein 0.2 g

Chili Powder, 1 tablespoon (8 g) is 22 kcal | total fat 1.1 g | carbs 4 g | fiber 2.8 g | protein 1.1 g

Cinnamon, 1 teaspoon is 6 kcal | total fat 0.07 g | carbs 2 g | fiber 1.4 g | protein 0.09 g

Cream of Tartar, 1 tablespoon is 7.7 kcal | total fat 0 g | carbs 1.8 g | fiber 0 g | protein 0 g

Cumin, Ground, 1 teaspoon is 11.3 kcal | total fat 0.7 g | carbs 1.3 g | fiber 0.3 g | protein 0.5 g

Dill, Fresh, 5 sprigs (1 g) is 0.4 kcal | total fat 0 g | carbs 0.1 g | fiber 0 g | protein 0 g

Garlic Powder, 1 teaspoon (3.1 g) is 10.3 kcal | total fat 0 g | carbs 2.3 g | fiber 0.3 g | protein 0.5 g

Garlic Salt, 1 teaspoon (5.6 g) is 4.8 kcal | total fat 0 g | carbs 1.1 g | fiber 0.1 g | protein 0.2 g

Horseradish, 1 tablespoon (5 g) is 5 kcal | total fat 0.1 g | carbs 1.19 g | fiber 0 g | protein 0.18 g

Hot Sauce, Original (Cholula), 1 teaspoon (4.7 g) is 0.5 kcal | total fat 0 g | carbs 0.1 g | fiber 0 g | protein 0 g

Onion Powder, 1 teaspoon (2.4 g) is 8.2 kcal | total fat 0.07 g | carbs 1.9 g | fiber 0.4 g | protein 0.3 g

Oregano, Leaves, 1 teaspoon (1 g) is 2.7 kcal | total fat 0 g | carbs 0.7 g | fiber 0.4 g | protein 0.1 g

Paprika, 1 teaspoon (2.3 g) is 6.5 kcal | total fat 0.27 g | carbs 1.2 g | fiber 0.8 g | protein 0.31 g

Parsley, 1 tablespoon (3.8 g) is 1.4 kcal | total fat 0.03 g | carbs 0.24 g | fiber 0.1 g | protein 0.11 g

Pepper, Black, 1 teaspoon (2.3 g) is 5.8 kcal | total fat 0.1 g | carbs 1.5 g | fiber 0.6 g | protein 0.2 g

Pumpkin Pie Spice, 1 teaspoon (1.7 g) is 5.8 kcal | total fat 0.21 g | carbs 1.2 g | fiber 0.3 g | protein 0.1 g

Salt (Morton), ⅓ teaspoon (1.5 g) is 0 kcal | total fat 0 g | carbs 0 g | fiber 0 g | protein 0 g

Salt, Coarse Kosher, ⅓ teaspoon (1.2 g) is 0 kcal | total fat 0 g | carbs 0 g | fiber 0 g | protein 0 g

Salt, Himalayan Pink (Olde Thompson), ⅓ teaspoon (1 g) is 0 kcal | total fat 0 g | carbs 0 g | fiber 0 g | protein 0 g

Salt, Sea (Morton), ⅓ teaspoon (1.5 g) is 0 kcal | total fat 0 g | carbs 0 g | fiber 0 g | protein 0 g

Turmeric, Ground, 1 teaspoon (3 g) is 9.4 kcal | total fat 0.1 g | carbs 2 g | fiber 0.7 g | protein 0.3 g

Sweeteners

Stevia, Granules, 0.8 teaspoon (3.5 g) is 0 kcal | total fat 0 g | carbs 3.5 g | fiber 0 g | protein 0 g

Stevia, Liquid, 1 teaspoon (7.1 g) is 0 kcal | total fat 0 g | carbs 2.3 g | fiber 0 g | protein 0 g

Swerve, Brown Sugar (Swerve), 1 teaspoon (4 g) is 0 kcal | total fat 0 g | carbs 4 g | fiber 0 g | protein 0 g

Swerve, Confectioners' (Powder) Sugar (Swerve), 1 teaspoon (5 g) is 0 kcal | total fat 0 g | carbs 5 g | fiber 0 g | protein 0 g

Swerve, Granular (Swerve), 1 teaspoon (3 g) is 0 kcal | total fat 0 g | carbs 3 g | fiber 0 g | protein 0 g

Vegetables

Shoppers may buy canned vegetables. I suggest reading the nutrition label on the packaging before buying to ensure that you aren't getting any hidden carbs, fillers, sodium (salt), or added sugars.

Artichoke, Hearts, ½ cup (130 g) is 35.1 kcal | total fat 0 g | carbs 6 g | fiber 4 g | protein 2 g

Asparagus, 5 spears (93 g) is 20 kcal | total fat 0 g | carbs 4 g | fiber 2 g | protein 2 g

Avocado, 1 serving (100 g) is 60 kcal | total fat 5 g | carbs 3 g | fiber 3 g | protein 1 g

Bean Sprouts, 1 serving (100 g) is 30 kcal | total fat 0 g | carbs 6 g | fiber 1 g | protein 3 g

Bell Peppers, Green, 1 medium (119 g) is 30 kcal | total fat 0.2 g | carbs 8 g | fiber 2 g | protein 1 g

Bell Peppers, Red, 1 medium (148 g) is 25 kcal | total fat 0.2 g | carbs 6 g | fiber 2 g | protein 1 g

Bok Choy (Chinese Cabbage), 3 ounces (84 g) is 10 kcal | total fat 0 g | carbs 2 g | fiber 1 g | protein 1 g

Broccoli, 5 ounces (141.75 g) is 43.1 kcal | total fat 0.5 g | carbs 7.7 g | fiber 2.9 g | protein 3.8 g

Brussel Sprouts, 1 serving (86 g) is 35 kcal | total fat 1.2 g | carbs 3.4 g | fiber 3.4 g | protein 2.9 g

Cabbage, Green, 5 ounces (141.75 g) is 116.7 kcal | total fat 8.3 g | carbs 10 g | fiber 3.3 g | protein 1.28 g

Carrot, 1 carrot (46 g) is 16 kcal | total fat 0.1 g | carbs 3.8 g | fiber 1.4 g | protein 0.3 g

Cauliflower, 1 cup (91 g) is 25 kcal | total fat 0.1 g | carbs 4 g | fiber 1 g | protein 1 g

Celery, 1 stalk of medium (7-½" to 8" long or 2 ounces) (56.7 g) is 8.5 kcal | total fat 0 g | carbs 2.3 g | fiber 1.1 g | protein 0 g

Cucumbers (Sliced with Peel), ½ cup or 2 ounces (56.7 g) is 8.5 kcal | total fat 0 g | carbs 1.7 g | fiber 0.6 g | protein 0.6 g

Eggplant, 1 cup cubed or 3.53 ounces (100 g) is 20 kcal | total fat 0.16 g | carbs 5 g | fiber 3 g | protein 1 g

Green String Beans, 1 cup (85 g) is 25 kcal | total fat 0 g | carbs 5 g | fiber 3 g | protein 1 g

Greens, Mustard, 1 serving (85 g) is 20 kcal | total fat 0 g | carbs 4 g | fiber 3 g | protein 2 g

Lettuce, Iceberg, 1 cup shredded or chopped (226.8 g) is 8 kcal | total fat 0.08 g | carbs 1.6 g | fiber 0.8 g | protein 0.4 g

Lettuce, Romaine, Chopped, 1 cup (45.36 g) is 5 kcal | total fat 0 g | carbs 1 g | fiber 1 g | protein 0.5 g

Mushrooms, Baby Bella Sliced, 3 ounces (85 g) are 20 kcal | total fat 0 g | carbs 2 g | fiber 1 g | protein 3 g

Mushrooms, Portabella Caps, 1 cap (85 g) is 20 kcal | total fat 0 g | carbs 3 g | fiber 1 g | protein 3 g

Mushrooms, White Button, Packaged, ⅓ cup or 5 medium shrooms (84 g) is 20 kcal | total fat 0 g | carbs 3 g | fiber 1 g | protein 3 g

Napa Cabbage, Shredded, 1 cup (76 g) is 15 kcal | total fat 0 g | carbs 2 g | fiber 1 g | protein 1 g

Okra, 1 cup or 3 ounces (85 g) is 33 kcal | total fat 0.9 g | carbs 5.3 g | fiber 2.7 g | protein 2.4 g

Olives, Black, Organic Pitted Kalamata, 4 olives (7 g) are 21 kcal | total fat 2.1 g | net carbs 0.5 g | fiber 0 g | protein 0 g

Olives, Organic Jumbo Green, 3 olives (15 g) are 25 kcal | total fat 2.5 g | carbs 1 g | fiber 0 g | protein 0 g

Onions, Green Chopped, ¼ cup (100 g) is 10 kcal | total fat 0 g | carbs 2 g | fiber 1 g | protein 0 g

Onions, Sweet, 1.5 ounces (100 g) are 10 kcal | total fat 0.02 g | carbs 1.84 g | fiber 0 g | protein 0.23 g

Onions, Yellow, ½ cup chopped (100 g) is 31 kcal | total fat 0 g | carbs 8.1 g | fiber 2 g | protein 0.7 g

Pepper, Banana, 1 small (4" long) (30 g) is 10 kcal | total fat 0 g | carbs 2 g | fiber 0 g | protein 0 g

Pepper, Hot Chili, 1 pepper (45 g) is 18 kcal | total fat 0.2 g | carbs 4. g | fiber 0.7 g | protein 0.8 g

Pepper, Poblano, 1 pepper (64 g) is 13 kcal | total fat 0.11 g | carbs 3 g | fiber 1.1 g | protein 0.55 g

Pepper, Serrano, 1 pepper (6.1 g) is 2 kcal | total fat 0.03 g | carbs 0.4 g | fiber 0.2 g | protein 0.11 g

Pepper, Sweet Red, 1 pepper (114 g) is 32 kcal | total fat 0.2 g | carbs 7.6 g | fiber 1.4 g | protein 1 g

Pickle, Dill, 1 spear (35 g) is 4.2 kcal | total fat 0.1 g | carbs 0.8 g | fiber 0.3 g | protein 0.2 g

Radish, 1 radish, medium (4.5 g) is 0.7 kcal | total fat 0 g | carbs 0.1 g | fiber 0.1 g | protein 0 g

Sauerkraut, Cooked, 1 cup is 27 kcal | total fat 0.2 g | carbs 6.1 g | fiber 4.1 g | protein 1.29 g

Snow Peas or Sugar Snap Peas, 1 cup (160 g) is 67 kcal | total fat 0.4 g | carbs 11 g | fiber 4.5 g | protein 5.2 g

Soybeans, 1 cup (172 g) is 296 kcal | total fat 15 g | carbs 14 g | fiber 10 g | protein 31 g

Spaghetti Squash, Cooked, 1 cup (100 g) is 47 kcal | total fat 2.56 g | carbs 6.3 g | fiber 1.4 g | protein 0.64 g

Spinach, Cooked from Fresh, 1 cup (180 g) is 41 kcal | total fat 0.5 g | carbs 6.8 g | fiber 4.3 g | protein 5.3 g

Spinach, Fresh Organic Baby, 1 cup (30 g) is 7 kcal | total fat 0 g | carbs 1.1 g | fiber 0.7 g | protein 0.9 g

Yellow Summer Squash, 1 cup sliced (approx. 175 g) is 18 kcal | total fat 0.2 g | carbs 3.79 g | fiber 1.2 g | protein 1.37 g

Zucchini, 1 medium (217 g) is 33 kcal | total fat 0.8 g | carbs 5.8 g | fiber 2.2 g | protein 2.5 g

Keto Substitutes for High Carb Foods

Substitute Mashed Cauliflower for Mashed Potatoes. Compare the following nutritional facts.

Mashed Cauliflower, 1 cup (228 g) is 204 kcal | total fat 17 g | carbs 9.8 g | fiber 4.6 g | protein 6.5 g

Mashed Potatoes, 1 cup (210 g) is 237 kcal | total fat 8.8 g | carbs 36 g | fiber 3.2 g | protein 4.1 g

Substitute Cauliflower rice for white or brown rice. Compare the following nutritional facts.

Cauliflower Rice, 1 cup (100 g) is 25 kcal | total fat 0.3 g | carbs 5 g | fiber 2 g | protein 1.9 g

Brown Rice, ½ cup (98 g) is 109 kcal | total fat 0.8 g | carbs 23 g | fiber 1.8 g | protein 2.3 g

White Rice, ½ cup (54 g) is 190 kcal | total fat 0 g | carbs 43 g | fiber 0 g | protein 4 g

Spiralized Zucchini for pasta noodles. Compare the following nutritional facts.

Zucchini, Noodles (Spiralized), 1 cup (118 g) is 20 kcal | total fat 0.4 g | carbs 3.7 g | fiber 1.2 g | protein 1.4 g

Pasta Noodles, 1 cup (spaghetti not packed) (124 g) is 196 kcal | total fat 1.2 g | carbs 38 g | fiber 2.2 g | protein 7.2 g

What Foods to Minimize

The following list is alphabetized for easy read and convenience. This list contains the serving size, calories (kcal), total fat, net carbs (total carbs minus fiber), and protein.

Note this list is for the Keto dieters following the Cyclical Keto Diet (CKD) and Targeted Keto Diet (TKD) or those who need more carbs per serving. These items contain more than 7 grams of net carbs.

If you wish to indulge in these items but don't want the carbs, consider reducing the serving size. For example, eat 1/2 of an apple instead of the whole apple. If you are following the Standard Keto Diet (SKD), you may eat these foods every once in a while. Don't eat them daily if you are trying to reverse diabetes or some other health condition that thrives on high carbs.

Remember carbs from this list are considered good carbs, which is different than on What Foods to Avoid list.

The nutritional facts are estimated and provided as a courtesy. The nutritional facts are generated by an online API which recognizes ingredient names and amounts and makes calculations from the serving size with algorithms. Results may vary.

Sources: nutritionix.com, carb manager app, or fatsecret.com.

Fruits

Apple, 1 medium 3-inch diameter (182 g) is 95 kcal | total fat 0.3 g | carbs 25 g | fiber 4.4 g | protein 0.5 g

Banana, 1 medium 7 to 7-⅞ inches long (118 g) is 105 kcal | total fat 0.4 g | carbs 27 g | fiber 3.1 g | protein 1.3 g

Date, 1 date, pitted (7.1 g) is 20 kcal | total fat 0 g | carbs 5.3 g | fiber 0.6 g | protein 0.2 g

Fig, 1 medium fig (2-¼ inch diameter) (50 g) is 37 kcal | total fat 0.1 g | carbs 9.6 g | fiber 1.5 g | protein 0.4 g

Grapefruit, ½ medium (123 g) is 52 kcal | total fat 0.2 g | carbs 13 g | fiber 2 g | protein 0.9 g

Grape, 10 grapes (49 g) are 34 kcal | total fat 0.1 g | carbs 8.9 g | fiber 0.4 g | protein 0.4 g

Guava, 1 cup, raw (165 g) is 112 kcal | total fat 1.6 g | carbs 24 g | fiber 8.9 g | protein 4.2 g

Kiwi Fruit, 1 medium fruit, 2-inch diameter (69 g) is 42 kcal | total fat 0.4 g | carbs 10 g | fiber 2.1 g | protein 0.8 g

Mango, 1 fruit without refuse, (336 g) is 202 kcal | total fat 1.3 g | carbs 50 g | fiber 5.4 g | protein 2.8 g

Melon (Muskmelon/Cantaloupes), 1 medium (about 5-inch diameter) (552 g) is 188 kcal | total fat 1 g | carbs 45 g | fiber 5 g | protein 4.6 g

Nectarine, 1 fruit (2-3/4-inch diameter) (156 g) is 69 kcal | total fat 0.5 g | carbs 16 g | fiber 2.7 g | protein 1.7 g

Orange, 1 small (2-7/8-inch diameter) (140 g) is 69 kcal | total fat 0.2 g | carbs 18 g | fiber 3.1 g | protein 1.3 g

Papaya, 1 cup 1-inch pieces (145 g) is 62 kcal | total fat 0.4 g | carbs 16 g | fiber 2.5 g | protein 0.7 g

Peach, 1 large (2-3/4-inch diameter) (175 g) is 68 kcal | total fat 0.4 g | carbs 17 g | fiber 2.6 g | protein 1.6 g

Pear, 1 medium (178 g) is 101 kcal | total fat 0.3 g | carbs 27 g | fiber 5.5 g | protein 0.6 g

Pineapple, ½ cup, chunks (83 g) is 41 kcal | total fat 0.1 g | carbs 11 g | fiber 1.2 g | protein 0.5 g

Plums, 1 fruit (2-⅛ inch diameter) (66 g) is 30 kcal | total fat 0.2 g | carbs 7.5 g | fiber 0.9 g | protein 0.5 g

Pomegranate, 1 fruit (4-inch diameter) (282 g) is 234 kcal | total fat 3.3 g | carbs 53 g | fiber 11 g | protein 4.7 g

Tangerine, 1 medium (2-½ inch diameter) (88 g) is 40 kcal | total fat 0.3 g | carbs 12 g | fiber 1.6 g | protein 0.7 g

Nuts & Seeds

(If you eat too many nuts, it can kick you out of ketosis)

Almonds, Raw, 10 almonds are 70 kcal | total fat 6.1 g | carbs 2.4 g | fiber 0.1 g | protein 2.6 g

Brazil Nuts, Raw, ¼ cup or 12 nuts (30 g) are 200 kcal | total fat 20 g carbs 4 g | fiber 2 g | protein 4 g

Cashews, Raw Whole, ⅛ cup (15 g) are 90 kcal | total fat 6.5 g | carbs 4.5 g | fiber 0.5 g | protein 3.5 g

Macadamia Nuts, 1 ounce or 10 to 12 nuts are 204 kcal | total fat 21.48 g | net carbs 3.92 g | fiber 2.4 g | protein 2.24 g

Peanuts, Dry Roasted, Unsalted, 10 nuts are 60 kcal | total fat 5 g | net carbs 2.1 g | protein 2.4 g

Peanuts, In Shell (Shell not eaten), 1 cup edible yield is 305 kcal | total fat 26.78 g | carbs 7.78 g | fiber 4.8 g | protein 14.3 g

Pecans, Chopped, ¼ cup (28 g) is 200 kcal | total fat 20 g | carbs 4 g | fiber 3 g | protein 3 g

Pecans, Halves, ¼ cup (28 g) is 190 kcal | total fat 20 g | carbs 4 g | fiber 3 g | protein 3 g

Pecans, Raw, ¼ cup (30 g) is 210 kcal | total fat 21 g | carbs 4 g | fiber 2 g | protein 3 g

Pistachio Nuts, 1 ounce or 49 kernels are 158 kcal | total fat 12.6 g | carbs 7.93 g | fiber 2.9 g | protein 5.84 g

Pumpkin Seeds, Raw, ¼ cup (30 g) is 170 kcal | total fat 15 g | carbs 3 g | fiber 2 g | protein 9 g

Sunflower Seeds, Raw, ¼ cup (30 g) is 170 kcal | total fat 15 g | carbs 6 g | fiber 3 g | protein 7 g

Sunflower Seeds, In Shell, 1 package (95 g) is 180 kcal | total fat 15 g | carbs 4 g | fiber 3 g | protein 6 g

Walnuts, Organic, ¼ cup (28 g) is 180 kcal | total fat 17 g | carbs 5 g | fiber 1 g | protein 4 g

Vegetables

Bell Peppers, Orange, 1 pepper (114 g) is 32 kcal | total fat 0.2 g | carbs 7.6 g | fiber 1.4 g | protein 1 g

Bell Peppers, Yellow, 1 large (186 g) is 50 kcal | total fat 0.4 g | carbs 12 g | fiber 1.7 g | protein 1.9 g

Onions, Red, 1 medium (94 g) is 41 kcal | total fat 0.2 g | carbs 9.5 g | fiber 1.3 g | protein 1.3 g

Peas, 1 cup (160 g) is 134 kcal | total fat 0.3 g | carbs 25 g | fiber 8.8 g | protein 2.3 g

What Foods to Avoid

As previously mentioned, the following lists provide a reference of foods to avoid. If you do eat any of these foods, don't eat them on a daily or regular basis.

The nutritional facts are estimated and provided as a courtesy. The nutritional facts are generated by an online API which recognizes ingredient names and amounts and makes calculations from the serving size with algorithms. Results may vary.

Sources: nutritionix.com, carb manager app, or fatsecret.com.

Artificial Sweeteners

Avoid artificial sweeteners such as Saccharin, sucralose (Splenda), aspartame. These sweeteners are not only bad for the body but also make you crave other simple sugars (Betsch, 2015).

Unfortunately, you find these artificial sweeteners, Saccharin or aspartame, in diet soda. Before, starting Keto, I was a diet soda fiend. I consumed, on the average, one 2-liter diet soda per day. Then I thought I would make a smart move and drink sparkling water instead of soda. Guess what? The sparkling water contains sucralose. Therefore, I exchanged my apple for an orange, so to speak. After discovering that, I changed to filtered water, and if I needed flavor, I added a fresh lemon or a lime. I feel better for this change.

However, I'll tell you that this was a tough switch for me because I loved…loved…loved…my diet soda and my sparkling water.

Now, I no longer have those wild food cravings for high carbs as I once did. I never knew that these added sweeteners were working behind the scenes to sabotage my weight loss strategy. If you're like me, this news comes as an eye-opening surprise.

Legumes

Beans, 1 cup (254 g) is 239 kcal | total fat 0.9 g | carbs 54 g | fiber 10 g | protein 12 g

Chickpeas, 1 cup (164 g) is 269 kcal | total fat 4.2 g | carbs 45 g | fiber 12 g | protein 15 g

Lentils, 1 cup (198 g) is 230 kcal | total fat 0.8 g | carbs 40 g | fiber 16 g | protein 18 g

Milk Products

Milk, 1 cup (245 g) is 125 kcal | total fat 4.7 g | carbs 12 g | fiber 0 g | protein 8.5 g

Processed Foods

Candy, (Hershey Chocolate Bar), 1 bar (43 g) is 220 kcal | total fat 13 g | carbs 26 g | fiber 1 g | protein 3 g

Corn Meal, 1 cup (122 g) is 442 kcal | total fat 4.4 g | carbs 94 g | fiber 8.9 g | protein 9.9 g

Flour, 1 cup (125 g) is 455 kcal | total fat 1.2 g | carbs 95 g | fiber 3.4 g | protein 13 g

Pre-Packaged or Prepared Foods

Soda Regular, 1 can or bottle (12 fluid ounces) (370 g) is 155 kcal | total fat 0.9 g | carbs 38 g | fiber 0 g | protein 0 g

Soda Diet, 1 can or bottle (12 fluid ounces) (355 g) is 7.1 kcal | total fat 0.1 g | carbs 1 g | fiber 0 g | protein 0.4 g (contains sucralose)

Sugar, 1 tablespoon (12.6 g) is 48 kcal | total fat 0 g | carbs 12.6 g | fiber 0 g | protein 0 g

Starchy Vegetables

Corn, 1 ear medium (103 g) is 99 kcal | total fat 1.5 g | carbs 22 g | fiber 2.5 g | protein 3.5 g

Potato, 1 medium (173 g) is 161 kcal | total fat 0.2 g | carbs 37 g | fiber 3.8 g | protein 4.3 g

Sweet Potato, 1 medium (2-inch diameter, 5-inches long) (114 g) is 103 kcal | total fat 0.2 g | carbs 24 g | fiber 3.8 g | protein 2.3 g

Yam, 1 cup, cubes (136 g) is 158 kcal | total fat 0.2 g | carbs 37 g | fiber 5.3 g | protein 2 g

Whole Grain Foods

Amaranth, 1 cup (246 g) is 251 kcal | total fat 3.9 g | carbs 46 g | fiber 5.2 g | protein 9.3 g

Barley, 1 cup (157 g) is 193 kcal | total fat 0.7 g | carbs 44 g | fiber 6 g | protein 3.5 g

Bread, Wheat, 1 slice (29 g) is 77 kcal | total fat 0.9 g | carbs 14 g | fiber 1.2 g | protein 3.1 g

Bread, White, 1 slice (29 g) is 77 kcal | total fat 1 g | carbs 14 g | fiber 0.8 g | protein 2.6 g

Breakfast cereals, (Cheerios), 1 cup (28 g) is 105 kcal | total fat 1.9 g | carbs 21 g | fiber 2.6 g | protein 3.4 g

Breakfast cereals, (Frosted Flakes), 1 cup (42 g) is 155 kcal | total fat 0.7 g | carbs 37 g | fiber 0.9 g | protein 1.7 g

Oatmeal, 1 cup (234 g) is 166 kcal | total fat 3.6 g | carbs 28 g | fiber 4 g | protein 5.9 g

Pasta Noodles, 1 cup (spaghetti not packed) (124 g) is 196 kcal | total fat 1.2 g | carbs 38 g | fiber 2.2 g | protein 7.2 g

Quinoa, ½ cup (93 g) is 111 kcal | total fat 1.8 g | carbs 20 g | fiber 2.6 g | protein 4.1 g

Brown Rice, ½ cup (98 g) is 109 kcal | total fat 0.8 g | carbs 23 g | fiber 1.8 g | protein 2.3 g

White Rice, ½ cup (54 g) is 190 kcal | total fat 0 g | carbs 43 g | fiber 0 g | protein 4 g

What Foods to Stock

Stock the following food items in your pantry. Start or build a supply of items for your keto recipes. Also, stock items from What Foods to Eat. Note the expiration date or if the item is perishable like some vegetables or fruit to minimize waste. Be sure to read the nutrition label to avoid unnecessary ingredients and added sugars or artificial sweeteners.

Source: nutritionix.com, carb manager app, or fatsecret.com. Nutrition information may vary.

Condiments

Mayonnaise is a good source of the good fat: serving size is 2 tablespoons.

Mustard: most mustards have zero carbs.

Hot sauce: some hot sauces are zero to one carb per tablespoon. I use the Siracha sauce to give my dishes enough fire and kick.

Salad Dressing: find a full-fat salad dressing that is not sweetened with sugar or artificial sweeteners with little or no carbs. Light salad dressing removes the fat and replace it with sugar. Don't buy light. Remember, the full fat contains the good fat. It's better for nutritional or optimal ketosis.

Flour and Thickeners

These flours are high fiber, low carb alternative to all-purpose flour. These flours bake well in the oven for Keto cookies or fry for Keto pancakes or waffles. These flours also thicken soups, sauces, and stews.

Almond flour: Has a great nutty flavor.

Almond meal: Great to use instead of bread crumbs or bread coating when frying.

Coconut flour: I use this flour to thicken the coconut oil and coconut butter in fat bombs, and I use this flour with the almond flour when baking.

Guar gum: Great for thickening soups, sauces, or stews.

Xanthum gum: Great for thickening soups, sauces, or stews.

Ghee

Ghee or clarified butter incorporates a rich nuttiness not found in everyday butter. Use to pan-fry vegetables or meats. If you are running low on your daily fat intake, you can eat a tablespoon of Ghee, which contains less calories than olive or coconut oil.

Nut Butters

These butters are the base for most fat bombs, smoothies, and as a dip for vegetables. These butters also are a good source for good fats. Find these butters with little or no sugar and fewest carbs.

- Almond Butter (Unsweetened)

- Peanut Butter (Unsweetened)

- Walnut Butter (Unsweetened)

Nuts and Seeds

These nuts and seeds are good source for good fats. Eat in moderation to minimize the calorie intake.

- Almonds

- Macadamia nuts

- Pecans

- Pumpkin seeds

- Sunflower Seeds

Oils

MCT oil: Derived from coconut and palm kernel oils. These saturated fatty acids are used and burned by your body instead of being stored. MCT oil helps keep your body functioning as a fat-burning machine.

Coconut oil: Great for frying, adding to coffee, or blending into a smoothie. It can be a lotion and moisturizer for dry skin. Many of the fat bomb recipes call for solid coconut oil. It tastes slightly sweet.

Coconut butter: Great for fat bomb recipes. It also tastes slightly sweet.

Cooking oils: Avocado oil, sunflower seed oil, and grapeseed oil have high smoke points. Great for sautéing, roasting, and stir-frying. These oils also have a neutral taste to be used in baking.

Non-cooking oils: Flaxseed oil, pistachio oil, and walnut oil are not cooking oils because they break down and burn quickly. These oils are great for drizzling over salads, adding to soups, or avocado dips.

Olives

Green and Black Olives are plentiful in heart-healthy fats. Add 3 to 6 olives to meals or snacks to increase your good fat intake.

Salt and Spices

Salt can ease the symptoms of the Keto flu. Spices are good. Check the ingredients label to ensure no hidden surprises such as additives or fillers. The Keto diet is actually a low-salt diet.

Sweeteners

Stevia is made from a South American plant called stevia. The leaves are 200 to 400 times sweeter than regular table sugar. The body does not absorb this sweetener; therefore, it passes through the body without affecting blood sugar.

Swerve is made from three ingredients: erythritol, oligosaccharides and natural flavor. The erythritol is made by fermenting glucose with a microorganism in brewery tanks, similar to the way that beer and wine are made. The natural flavors are added to replicate the taste of table sugar. The body also does not absorb this sweetener, and it passes through the body without affecting the blood sugar.

Keto Supplements

One side effect of the Keto diets is dehydration or depletion of electrolytes and/or minerals. It is important to drink plenty of water, and the following supplements may help you retain or replenish electrolytes and/or minerals. However, each supplement contains its own advantages and disadvantages.

I provide you with my own experience with each of these supplements to help you decide if these supplements are right for you. At the time of this writing, Beta-Hydroxybutyrate (BHB) and Medium Chain Triglycerides (MCT) Oil are popular among Keto dieters. I examine these supplements and others to give you a complete scenario. I summarized the following supplements from my research findings from Drs. Phinney's and Volek's (2018) blog.

Beta-Hydroxybutyrate (BHB)

The body produces BHB ketones, naturally, when you are in ketosis, from fat in the liver for energy when glucose is no longer available. These ketones become the body's primary source of energy. Sometimes the body needs a boost of BHB from external or outside sources, and that is where this supplement helps: the BHB supplement is an exogenous ketone supplement.

Advantages

- Reach ketosis quicker

- Alleviates Keto flu symptoms

- Reduces hunger and eliminates cravings

- Improves energy levels and mental performance

- Increases physical performance and longer lasting energy

- Starts the fat burning process making the body a fat burning machine

- Decreases stress and fatigue

Disadvantages

- Short-lived benefits

- Ingested ketones become waste if the body doesn't need them

- Adds extra calories to diet

- Unpleasant taste in some of the flavors available

- Shuts down the fat burning process if supplement is taken daily for an extended period

- May have excessive price rendering this supplement an uneconomical choice

- May cause diarrhea or constipation

The BHB supplement is for the smart beginner who wants to achieve ketosis faster or alleviate the Keto flu symptoms or for the athlete or body builder who needs improved energy and physical stamina. If you take this supplement for an extended period, it may slow or stall your weight loss progress. Be sure the BHB supplement contains equal to less than 2 net carbs per serving.

Electrolytes

Electrolytes are chemicals conducting electricity when mixed with water. The following list shows which electrolytes are eliminated by the body and must be replaced to make the body function properly:

- Calcium

- Chloride

- Magnesium

- Phosphorus

- Potassium

- Sodium

Advantages

- Improves exercise performance

- Replenishes water

- Helps recover energy

- Rehydrates during illness

- Prevents heat stroke

- Regulates nerve and muscle function

- Balances blood acidity and pressure

- Rebuilds damaged tissue

Disadvantages

The following disadvantages are the results of increased or decreased levels of electrolytes (potassium, magnesium, sodium, or calcium) in the blood causing:

- Convulsions

- Dizziness or confusion

- Fast or irregular heartbeat

- High blood pressure

- Irritability

- Muscle twitching

- Restlessness

- Swelling of feet or lower legs

- Bone disorders

Keto Shake

Several companies offer a Keto shake as a meal replacement. I drink the Keto Function Keto + Shake Dutch Chocolate as a meal replacement for breakfast and sometimes dinner. I mix the powder supplement with 1 cup of Almond Milk and 1 cup of Water. It tastes almost like the chocolate milk that I drank as a child. This supplement contains caffeine, which helps your body stay in ketosis. If you are sensitive to caffeine, it may not be for you.

Advantages

- Reduces hunger and eliminates cravings.

- Improves energy levels and mental alertness.

- Helps the body stay in ketosis; however, you can still kick yourself out of ketosis if you consume too many high carbs or sugary foods or drinks.

- Contains some of the need electrolytes and minerals.

- Tastes good depending on brand and flavor.

Disadvantages

- May cause diarrhea or constipation if sensitive to ingredients. Check the ingredients to ensure that it helps you stay on your diet regimen.

- May have excessive price rendering this supplement an uneconomical choice. Try with dark cocoa

L-Theanine

L-Theanine is an enzyme found in black or green tea. It is safe to consume if you don't overdo it.

Advantages

- Improves metal focus

- Helps with relaxation and sleep

- Increases mental performance

- Enhances weight loss

- Boosts the immune system

- Reduces blood pressure

- Supports the performance of certain cancer drugs

Disadvantages

- May cause upset stomach if overconsumed

- May cause irritability from caffeine if sensitive

Magnesium

Magnesium is a mineral and electrolyte abundant in the body. The foods containing magnesium are nuts and spinach. The body discards excessive magnesium through perspiration, dehydration, and waste, and some medicines rid the body of magnesium as a side effect. The recommended dosage is 350 mg daily. Anyone with a kidney disorder should not take magnesium with consulting their personal doctor or healthcare provider.

The body absorbs several types of magnesium supplements:

- Aspartate
- Chloride
- Citrate
- Glycinate
- Lactate

Advantages

- Increased energy
- Better sleep
- Reduced muscle aches
- Improved heart health
- Controlled migraines
- Improved digestion and muscles in the digestive tract including the intestinal wall
- Counterbalances stomach acid
- Advances stools through the intestines
- Helps the heart maintain a healthy rhythm
- Regulates blood pressure and production of cholesterol
- Reduces cardiovascular disease
- Helps with food metabolism
- Helps the body with nerve signal transmission

- Balances fluids

- Maintains bone and muscle health

Disadvantages

The following disadvantages are from taking a magnesium supplement in high doses may cause:

- Diarrhea (if overconsumed)

- Kidney problems

- Low blood pressure

- Urine retention

- Nausea and vomiting

- Depression and lethargy

- Slowed breathing

- Loss of central nervous system (CNS) control

- Cardiac arrest or irregular heartbeat

- Coma or death

Medium Chain Triglyceride (MCT) Oil

MCT oil supplement is a type of fatty acid found in coconut oil. Naturally, the liver metabolizes these fats transforming them into a fuel source. Everyone on the Keto diets should take this supplement.

Advantages

- Contains magnesium, electrolytes, and fiber

- Increases the metabolism

- Reduces food cravings and hunger

- Helps dieters achieve good fat ratio

- Increases the effectiveness of the Keto diet

- Helps to relieve the Keto flu

Disadvantages

- May cause stomach cramps or aches

- May cause constipation or diarrhea

- May not dissolve completely

MCT Oil supplement is for the smart beginner or seasoned pro who wants to increase their electrolytes, magnesium, fiber, and good fat ratios. Even though this supplement may contain a few disadvantages such as stomach upset, diarrhea, or constipation, it helps the dieter stop hunger cravings and stay full longer.

MCT Oil supplement is available in powder and liquid forms. Be sure the MCT Oil supplement contains equal to less than 2 net carbs per serving.

Minerals

If you take a multi vitamin containing minerals such as Calcium, Copper, Iodine, Iron, Magnesium, Manganese, Molybdenum, Nickel, Pantothenic Acid, Phosphorus, Potassium, Selenium, Sodium Chloride, and Zinc, you are already getting your daily requirement. Be sure to follow the recommended dosage listed on the packaging.

Advantages

- Build strong teeth and bones

- Control body fluids in cells

- Turns food into energy

- Transmits nerve impulses

Disadvantages (if taken in overdose)

- Nausea

- Diarrhea

- Stomach cramps

- Hair loss

- Gastrointestinal upset

- Fatigue

- Mild nerve damage

Multi-Vitamin

Several good multi-vitamins are available providing the daily requirement for Vitamin A, B1 (Thiamin), B2 (Riboflavin), B3 (Niacin), B6 (Pyridoxine), B9 (Folic Acid), B12, C, D, E, K, minerals, and so on. Be sure to following the recommended dosage.

Advantages

- Lower risk of heart disease

- Reduce risk of cancer

- Improves mood and cognition

- Promotes healthy skin (Vitamin C and D)

- Boost immune system

Disadvantages

- May interact with prescription medication

- Can become toxic at high dosages

Omega-3 Fatty Acids

Omega-3 fatty acids are found in fish oil supplements. Many health benefits are associated with Omega-3 fatty acids. Be sure to following the recommended dosage.

Advantages

- Fights depression and anxiety

- Improves eye health

- Promotes brain health during pregnancy and early life

- Reduces risk of heart disease

- Reduces symptoms of metabolic syndrome

- Increases blood circulation

Disadvantages

- Increases blood sugar

- Reduces coagulation

- May cause diarrhea

- May cause acid reflux

- Increases chance of stroke

- Increases chance of Vitamin A toxicity

- May cause insomnia

Probiotic

Probiotics are live microbes that are ingested through food supplements. Be sure to follow the recommended dosage.

Advantages

- Promotes good bacteria in the digestive system
- Prevent and treat diarrhea
- Improve mental health conditions
- Promotes heart health
- Reduces severity of certain allergies and eczema
- Reduces severity of inflammatory bowel disease
- Boost immune system
- Promotes losing weight and losing belly fat

Disadvantages

- Increase in gas and bloating
- May cause constipation
- Increase chance of dehydration
- May cause headaches
- May cause allergies to milk sugar or lactose
- May cause sensitivity to infection

Turmeric

Turmeric is a plant-derived antioxidant supplement, great for reducing inflammation. Be sure to following the recommended dosage.

Advantages

- May prevent heart disease, Alzheimer's, and cancer

- Reduces inflammation

- Reduces symptoms of depression and arthritis

Disadvantages

- May cause upset stomach, nausea, and diarrhea

- May cause dizziness

- May cause abnormal heart rhythm (if taken at high dosage)

Apple Cider Vinegar

Apple Cider Vinegar is not a Keto supplement, per se. I included it in my Keto regimen because of its natural healing and remedy properties. I provide the following summary from the article, "6 Health Benefits of Apple Cider Vinegar, Backed by Science" (Gunnars, n.d.). I also provide my experience with consuming apple cider vinegar for the last six months.

The distillation process places the apples in vinegar for a certain period, and the apples ferment similar to the whiskey fermenting process. With the apple cider vinegar, the by-product from the fermenting process is the acetic acid. This acid is what gives the apple cider vinegar its healing or magical properties. However, not any apple cider vinegar will do.

You must buy the organic apple cider vinegar with <u>Mother</u>.

On appearance, the vinegar looks like it has some sort of brownish, dirt-like substance in the liquid. However, this substance is what makes the vinegar work.

For best results, take 1 to 2 tablespoons diluted in 16.9 fluid ounces (500 ml) of water or tea before bedtime.

I take this dosage every night since I started my Keto regimen. It works for me, and I am sure that it will work for you too. The taste takes a little time to get accustomed to, but the benefits are amazing. If it seems a little strong to the taste, I add a couple of drops of lemon and lime juice.

I recommend apple cider vinegar for those with type 2 diabetes. However, I do not recommend apple cider vinegar for those with Type 1 diabetes.

Advantages

- Kills many types of harmful bacteria

- Lowers blood sugar levels for those who have type 2 diabetes

- Fights diabetes

- Helps you lose weight

- Reduces belly fat

- Lowers cholesterol

- Improves heart health

- Fights obesity

- Treats dandruff, sore throats, and varicose veins

Disadvantages

- Damages teeth or throat if you take more than the recommend dosage

- Cause upset stomach

- Lowers potassium levels because it works as a diuretic

- Slows the rate of food and liquids moving out of the stomach and intestines in Type 1 diabetes

- Slows digestion making it harder to control blood sugar level in Type 1 diabetes

- May cause some medications not to work. Consult your doctor if you are taking a medication that may be incompatible with apple cider vinegar.

STEP 3
DEVELOP A WEIGHT LOSS STRATEGY

How Weight Loss Works

At one time in my life, I sought the help of nutritionists, to prepare a diet plan for me. One nutritionist told me that you have to make the three food groups work in concert with each other and against each other to make weight loss effective. At that time, I thought what kind of double talk is that? However, now I agree in part with her statement. The food groups must work with and against each other. For example, if you prepare vegetables, cook or steam one vegetable and eat the other vegetable raw without cooking. It sounds crazy, but it works.

Even though you learned how the food groups work under step 2, you must know that no magic formula exists for dieting. Like with any diet, you can still gain weight on a Keto diet if you overeat. To make weight loss work, you must be aware of how many calories and carbs you consume, and you need to know what the maximum number of calories you need to lose weight. For me, at the beginning if I consumed less than 800 calories per day, I dropped two to five pounds per week, and I lost 30 pounds in 2 months on the Keto diet. I know part of this weight was water retention. However, my body did not store 30 pounds of water.

To be completely safe with losing weight, the average amount of weight that anyone should lose is approximately 2 pounds per week.

Keep in mind men lose weight faster than women. I know my female readers may be cursing or shooting lightning bolts at me, but ladies it's not my rule.

Calories are a key factor in losing weight at the beginning. After you are in the diet for a month or two, instinctively you will know how many calories and carbs you are consuming and counting them becomes less of a big deal.

You ask, what are calories and why should you count them?

Calories

A dictionary definition of calories mentions that it is "a unit of heat equal to the amount of heat needed to raise the temperature of one gram of water by one degree Celsius or 1.8 degrees Fahrenheit" (Definition of CALORIE, 2020). This unit measures the energy released by food as it is digested by the human body called calories (a.k.a. kilocalorie (kCal)).

Because of the Internet today, many calorie counters are available. Some counters are free, and some aren't. I describe these counter apps further in Tracking for Success.

Food scientists use a special counter requiring them to burn the food item to a crisp to determine the number of calories the item releases (Clarke, 2019; Jennings, 2020).

You don't have to burn your dinner to count calories. However, I encourage you to track carbs, calories, and weight to be successful on your Keto weight loss journey.

Smart beginners who track calories and carbohydrates are three times more successful than those who don't (Sifferlin, 2017). Therefore, tracking your calorie and carb consumption is the third step to your weight loss success.

Setting Goals

Setting weight loss goals can be intimidating. I summarized and rationalized the information in this section from research articles and from my own experience with setting weight loss goals (Herr, 2017; Migala, 2019).

A few years ago, about 15…to give a year or two, my wife and I participated in our first weight loss program. They asked us what weight we wanted as our end goal.

At that moment, I had no idea, and I picked a number out of the blue. That was my first mistake.

Even if the end weight goal is unknown, don't just grab a number. That number is what I call the big goal number. It's alright if you don't know what it is at the moment. With goal setting, you have two goals: a big goal number, and a little goal number. The little goal number is more important because it makes the difference between success and failure. I explain the little goal number further in the following subsections.

To be successful, the little number must be specific, measurable, attainable, realistic, and tangible to work in your weight loss strategy. Before looking at the goal definitions and specifics, establish a starting point.

The most important part of setting a goal is to know your starting point.

At the end of this chapter, see the section on taking your body measurements. Also step on the scale and record your starting weight. **These numbers are very important.**

Specific Goal

To set a specific goal, smart beginners assess their current weight condition. What is your current weight? What would you like your weight to be?

First, evaluate where you are starting.

A specific goal is to lose 10 pounds. By answering this question with a specific number, smart beginners attain their little number goal.

Let's say the smart beginners decide to lose 10 pounds. Let's analyze this goal further.

Measurable Goal

Smart beginners decide their little number goal is to lose 10 pounds. Is this number measurable? Yes. The average man loses about 2 pounds per week, and the average woman loses about 1.5 pounds per week. Your actual progress may be better or worse than the average. Again, I don't make the rules. Those facts, however, are sometimes true.

As you lose weight, you can calculate the results against the goal. Therefore, this goal is measurable.

Attainable Goal

Is losing 10 pounds attainable? Yes. After smart beginners get into their routine, they see the weight is coming off, and their attitude toward the diet becomes happier. You, too, will look forward to stepping on the scale every morning or twice a week, depending on how you want to track your progress. After you meet this goal, you see that it was very attainable.

By keeping the little number small and attainable, you will see each time you reset your goal that you will be able to knock out each level. After three to six weeks, you notice the big number goal is coming into focus as an attainable goal.

Realistic Goal

Is losing 10 pounds realistic? Ask yourself, is this goal too big or too small? If your little goal number is too big, you will give up trying because it becomes a huge number that looms out there in nowhere land. You don't want your number to end up being a fantasy or an albatross. You want your number to be realistic, and to do that, you must keep the number small enough to be attained in a week or in a few weeks. Don't be afraid to pick a smaller number like 5 pounds…or even 2 or 3 pounds.

A goal must have a time constraint. If smart beginners set a goal without a time constraint, they may get bored because the end goal is not visible. That was the second mistake I made when my wife and I went to the big-name weight loss program.

My wife and I got bored with the program. We made good progress, but we quit because we saw no end in sight. In fact, we made that mistake multiple times with other famous-name weight loss programs because the end goal was not visible, or we lost focus of it.

Set your little goal number at X pounds lost in Y number of days.

If the smart beginners set the number too small, they may get bored and give up because the process provides no challenge.

When I started Keto, my small number goal became 10 pounds per level. I call each goal a level for a frame of reference.

Tangible Goal

The definition of tangible is "to feel." Then, you must be able to feel your goal. You must be able to see your progress that you are making. The following recount of my experience fits in the Realistic Goal and the Tangible Goal section. I'm sure you will get the feeling of my goal setting from this recollection.

In August 15, 2019, my starting weight was at 254 pounds and the first number I wanted to attain was 250. I reached that number in about 4 days. My next little number goal was 10 pounds making my weight 240 pounds. I reached that number in about 2 to 3 weeks. The next goal was another 10 pounds making my weight 230 pounds and so on. As you see, I attained these goals because they were realistic and manageable. On November 15, 2019, I weighed 219 pounds before I saw my doctor. My doctor was ecstatic. I had lost 35 pounds in three months. I am half-way to my big number goal.

Little Number Goal

Now, you should have your little number goal in mind. It should be specific, measurable, realistic, and tangible.

Is the number too big or too small? Either way, it holds the keys to your success. Don't worry if you don't have a number in mind. After reading the chapter, Getting Started, you will have some goal in mind then.

Big Number Goal

To help smart beginners find their big number goal, they answer this question: **Why do you need to lose weight?** This "why" question is important and to answer it will help you attain your big number goal. Write your answer down. Some smart beginners keep journals, or they write it down on a piece of paper and put it in a safe place.

As previously mentioned, I needed to lose weight for health reasons. I picked 200 as my big goal number partially from what my doctor discussed with me. She said if I were to lose to 200, I could stop taking some of my medication. Even though that number seemed big, it is a good goal number to be looming off in the distance. I have an incentive to reach it because of the promise of better health. From my knowledge of goal setting in business, I know you need two goals: one goal is smaller and attainable, and the other goal is larger and abstract. This number seems to fit with this strategy.

Taking Your Body Measurements

Besides setting your weight loss goal, take your body measurements to attain a starting point. Experts advise you to take your best body measurements following these steps (Herr, 2017; Waehner, 2013):

1. Wear fitted clothing or no clothing.

2. Stand with your feet together and relax your body for all measurements.

3. Use a flexible, non-stretchy tape measure such as a cloth tape.

4. Take at least two measurements for chest, each arm (biceps), waist, hips, each thigh (upper legs), and each calf (lower legs).

Body	First measurement	Second measurement
Chest	_____________	_____________
L. Arm	_____________	_____________
R. Arm	_____________	_____________
Waist	_____________	_____________
Hip	_____________	_____________
L. Thigh	_____________	_____________
R. Thigh	_____________	_____________
L. Calf	_____________	_____________
R. Calf	_____________	_____________

5. Average each measurement; for example, measuring a woman's arms (biceps) first at 12.4 inches (31.5 cm) and second at 12.6 inches (32 cm), take the average measurement at 12.5 inches (31.75 cm).

Don't worry if you lose inches without losing weight at first. That's actually a good sign because you're losing fat and retaining or gaining muscle, especially if you're exercising or performing a workout routine.

Tracking for Success

Don't be afraid to track your food macronutrients and calories, and your weight. Smart beginners who track usually lose weight three times faster than those who do not (Sifferlin, 2017). After you notice some progress, logging every bite of food and stepping on the scale in the morning may not be such a burden after all. The following sections explain different tracking apps available.

The following steps recaps and summarizes earlier sections, to track for success, apply the following steps:

Step 1. Start prepared. Before starting, download a carb or calorie counting app or online tool or write down your calories, carbs, fats, proteins, and weight daily in a notebook. Then choose how to measure or estimate food portions before making a meal plan. You may only require a half portion compared to a full portion.

Step 2. Read food labels. Food labels comprise a lot of information for counting calories. Be sure to notice the portion size recommended on the package. Refer to Reading Nutrition Labels.

Step 3. Remove temptation. Rid your house pantry of all junk and high carb foods. By ridding the house of those foods, you won't be tempted to cheat on or abandon your diet.

Step 4. Go slow. Don't eliminate carbs or calories too fast. You may lose weight faster, but you may feel hunger pains, food withdrawals, or the Keto flu, making your diet success harder and running the risk of quitting.

Step 5. Drink plenty of water and eat enough food to include exercise. Successful weight loss programs include both diet and exercise. Drink at least eight 8-ounce (236 ml) glasses of water every day to stay hydrated. Keep your energy up so that you'll feel like exercising.

Tracking Carbs, Fat, Protein, and Fiber

Tracking carbs, fat, protein, and fiber is not as hard as it was a few years ago. With the invention of smart phones and apps, smart beginners can track everything from macronutrients to exercise to sleep to vital signs. Many of the carb tracking apps also track calories and weight. The following apps with the price and attributes are available at the time of this writing for download as described:

Carb Manager at https://www.carbmanager.com: this website and app offers a basic app for **FREE**, and a premium app for $3.34 per month billed annually. With the premium app you have the capability of tracking full nutrients, meal planner, track blood glucose, track ketones, track sleep, and have access to thousands of web Keto recipes and curated meal plans. This app allows you to track carbs, fat, protein, fiber, and so on.

Keto Diet Tracker at keto app (found in the Apple App Store or on Google Play): this app allows you to personalize macro goals, body type, and activity level. Use their search engine to input food and beverages and scan product barcodes. The search suggestions mark foods to avoid helping you maintain daily goals. It also has options for exercise and water tracking (Buckley, 2019).

Tracking Calories

The following steps will help you count calories and be successful with your ketogenic diet. The following calorie counting apps are available and current at the time of this writing:

My Fitness Pal at https://www.myfitnesspal.com/apps: this app offers a bunch of apps mostly for tracking fitness and exercise. This site also offers the Fitbit Tracker which allows you to track your weight, food, sleep, and exercise. The downside to the Fitbit Tracker requires owning a Fitbit watch.

Lose It! at https://www.loseit.com: this app offers a basic plan for **FREE**, but it does not do as much tracking as the premium plan for $3.33 per month. However, the basic plan allows you to track calories, exercise, community access, Apple Health and Google Fit sync, and Wi-Fi scale support.

Fat Secret at https://www.fatsecret.com: this app offers a food diary, healthy recipes, nutritional information, exercise diary, weight chart and journal, mobile apps for iPhone, iPad, Android, Blackberry, and Windows phones. This app is **FREE**, and it comes with a supportive community.

Cron-o-meter at https://cronometer.com: this app offers a **FREE** signup. The Cron-o-meter dashboard offers a diary, progress trends, foods, and profile. The website offers a blog, forums, and email.

Tracking Weight

If you don't have a weight scale, you may need one to track your weight. Many arguments state these scales are not accurate. However, these scales do offer a benchmark type number to compare your weight for tomorrow's weight against the weight from today and yesterday if you've written it down or recorded it in an app. Many of the apps as described above also allows you to enter your weight on a daily basis.

When I started, I weighed myself daily and recorded it. I saw the progress I made on a daily basis. I compared it with my weekly and monthly progress. I knew when I made good progress and when I hit a diet plateau. I learned what I must do to get past these obstacles. I still weigh myself daily.

By you tracking your food intake and weight, you will manage your progress better and easier during your Keto weight loss journey.

Developing a Meal Plan

Don't let the idea of creating a meal plan scare you. Soon you will become a seasoned pro at developing meal plans.

Be sure to make your meal plan flexible (Eenfeldt, 2018). Things happen without notice, and your plan should allow for guest popping in at the last minute without notice or working late at the office. Plan for consistency. If you can eat the same item day after day, all week long, this type of planning allows you to think about other things. If you cannot eat the same item day after day, plan for variety. A change in the menu can provide excitement without kicking you out of ketosis.

Most of all, make healthy keto friendly choices, and stick to your meal plan. Don't take a lot of time to prepare your meal plan, and then say, "I don't want that" or "I'm not feeling it" on the meal plan day. That type of thinking will cause your diet to fail.

To increase success with the Keto diet, develop a meal plan. A meal plan empowers you to develop a mindset after you:

- Create a grocery shopping list

- Look for nutritious keto friendly foods

- Stick to your food budget and diet

- See positive results

A meal plan also teaches you to manage in following manner:

- Save money and budget time

- Reduce grocery shopping trips

- Eliminate or minimizes impulse shopping

- Learn what to buy and prepare for meals

- Plan for leftovers

- Improve health by controlling portion sizes and food choices, and staying accountable

Make a meal plan for a few days or a couple of weeks to provide you with consistency, flexibility, and variety. With a meal plan, you make wiser choices when creating your shopping list, which saves you time and money.

Be sure to include the following details into your meal plan:

- Flexibility

- Consistency

- Variety

After a few weeks of making your meal plan, the process becomes second nature to you. A meal plan will help you stay on track with your Keto diet (Satterthwaite, 2018).

Developing an Exercise Plan

Start a regular exercise routine. Start slowly by taking little walks around the office or around the block. If you have a gym membership and are not applying it, start by going one day a week and working with one machine.

Don't start with the tread mill. Use one of the weight machines. Then increase your attendance to 2 days and use 2 machines. Stay off the tread mill until you are at least halfway to your big weight loss goal. Increase your attendance as you feel comfortable with and increase the usage of the machines.

It is always a good idea to ask a buddy to go with you to the gym. If you make an appointment to meet someone at the gym, you will be more likely to keep your date with the gym.

According to Gilson (2018), develop an exercise plan with

- Consistency – train the same day(s) each week. Write down an exercise schedule

- Active Recovery – most exercise plans allow one day to rest between exercise days. Perform a different type of less strenuous exercise on the recovery day

- Variety – change up your exercise routine to avoid boredom and exercise burnout

- Challenge – create an exercise program that will increase the number of workout routines and intensity, from easy to difficult over a certain time period

- Track Results – keep record of your exercise routines. Detail what you did correctly; what challenges you faced; and what you can do differently to improve or create variety and challenge

STEP 4
IMPLEMENT YOUR WEIGHT LOSS STRATEGY

Getting Started

Beginners Meal Plan

Intermediate Meal Plan

Advanced Meal Plan

Metabolic Reset

Energy & Exercise

Fasting

    Fasting Rules

    14-Hour Fasting

    18-Hour Fasting

    24-Hour Fasting

    Intermittent Fasting

Getting Started

Getting started on your weight loss journey can be scary. The unknown is often intimidating because you don't know the outcome. Some people, like me, will jump into the middle of a challenge without having all the facts and figure out the problems as they arrive. This type of action may be successful or unsuccessful, but that's part of the fun. Others may be a bit more cautious.

The ketogenic diet is more of a mindset than a physical diet. Others will say, "No! It's physical." However, if you have the mindset to begin, then the diet physicality is minimized. You have already succeeded. You have already won!

At the beginning of this book, I commented that you will have the foreknowledge of my mistakes and my successes and will be able to fast forward your success to arrive at your weight goal quicker than I did.

To recap the previous chapters, you have read and learned the Keto process, how Keto works, and ketosis. You understand the food groups, how to read nutrition labels, what foods to eat, what foods to minimize, what foods to avoid, and what foods to stock in your pantry. You've developed a weight loss strategy, including setting a little number goal and a big number goal, and understand tracking carbs, calories, and weight. You also have the flexibility of not tracking too. You've developed a meal plan and an exercise plan.

Now, it's time to implement this knowledge into a weight loss strategy. Feel free to go back to any of the previous chapters and read or refresh your memory.

To get started on the standard ketogenic diet, keep the following points in mind (Holland, 2019):

- Keep your carb intake low. Strive for 20 grams or less daily, preferred for strict SKD; or definitely keep your carbs under 50 grams daily

- Eat enough good fats like avocados, nuts, coconut oil, and so on.). Keep your good fat intake at about 70 to 75 percent of your total calorie and gram intake

- Drink lots of water. The ketogenic diet may dehydrate you if you're not drinking enough water, about eight 8-ounce glasses (236 ml) of water daily

- Replenish your electrolytes through your diet or supplements

- Eat when hungry. Don't forget to eat snacks at 10 a.m., 2 p.m., and 7 p.m. By having a vegetable snack or fat bomb, it will keep you from feeling too hungry at the next meal. Don't let the clock tell you when to eat. If you're hungry at 11 a.m. or 5 p.m., don't wait. Have lunch or dinner at the time that you are hungry

- Eat foods that are low carb such as meats, good carb vegetables, avocados, nuts and so on

- Don't eat too much protein. Your protein intake should be about 20 to 25 percent of your total calorie and gram intake

- Develop and implement an exercise regimen. Start slow. If you're like me, you've enjoyed a sedentary lifestyle most of your life. Work into a regular exercise workout routine

Beginners Meal Plan

Eat this meal plan for 2 to 6 weeks. The following plan keeps your carbs to less than 30 grams daily and definitely less than 50 grams daily (Eenfeldt, 2018).

The following guidelines provides flexibility and variety, while supporting you with the foundational structure needed to choose Keto-friendly meals.

Breakfast:

Choose 1 breakfast dish for breakfast containing less than 7 grams of carbs. See breakfast recipes.

Day	Meal Item	Number of Calories/Carbs
Sun.		
Mon.		
Tues.		
Wed.		
Thurs.		
Fri.		
Sat.		

Snacks:

Choose 1 snack for morning (10 a.m.), afternoon (3 p.m.), and evening (7 p.m.) containing less than 7 grams of carbs daily. See snack recipes.

Day	Meal Item	Number of Calories/Carbs
Sun.		
Mon.		
Tues.		
Wed.		
Thurs.		
Fri.		
Sat.		

Lunch and Dinner:

Choose 1 lunch dish at 12 noon and 1 dinner dish at 6 p.m. containing less than 7 grams of carbs daily. See lunch and dinner recipes.

Day	Meal Item	Number of Calories/Carbs
Sun.		
Mon.		
Tues.		
Wed.		
Thurs.		
Fri.		
Sat.		

Intermediate Meal Plan

The Beginners Meal Plan is a prerequisite to this meal plan. Eat this meal plan for 4 to 6 weeks. The following plan keeps your carbs to less than 20 grams daily. Pick one day to fast from 12 to 18 hours (Eenfeldt, 2018).

The following guidelines provides flexibility and variety, while supporting you with the foundational structure needed to choose Keto-friendly meals.

Breakfast:

Choose 1 breakfast dish for breakfast containing less than 7 grams of carbs daily or choose a meal replacement drink. See breakfast recipes.

Day	Meal Item	Number of Calories/Carbs
Sun.		
Mon.		
Tues.		
Wed.		
Thurs.		
Fri.		
Sat.		

Snacks:

Choose 1 snack for morning at 10 a.m., 1 snack for afternoon at 3 p.m., and 1 snack for evening 7 p.m. containing less than 5 grams of carbs daily. See snack recipes.

Eliminate one snack every other day. For example: on Monday, Wednesday, and Friday, you will eat only two snacks instead of three.

Day	Meal Item	Number of Calories/Carbs
Sun.		
Mon.		
Tues.		
Wed.		
Thurs.		
Fri.		
Sat.		

Lunch and Dinner:

Choose 1 lunch dish at 12 noon and 1 dinner dish at 6 p.m. containing less than 7 grams of carbs. or choose a meal replacement drink unless you drank it earlier. See lunch and dinner recipes.

Day	Meal Item	Number of Calories/Carbs
Sun.		
Mon.		
Tues.		
Wed.		
Thurs.		
Fri.		
Sat.		

Advanced Meal Plan

Eat this meal plan for 4 to 6 weeks for a total of 12 to 16. The following plan keeps your carbs to less than 20 grams per day. Pick two to three days to fast 18 hours or pick one day to fast 24 hours (Eenfeldt, 2018).

The following guidelines provides flexibility and variety, while supporting you with the foundational structure needed to choose Keto-friendly meals.

Breakfast:

Choose 1 breakfast dish for breakfast containing less than 5 grams of carbs daily or choose a meal replacement drink. See breakfast recipes.

Day	**Meal Item**	**Number of Calories/Carbs**
Sun.		
Mon.		
Tues.		
Wed.		
Thurs.		
Fri.		
Sat.		

Snacks:

Choose 1 snack for afternoon (3 p.m.). containing less than 5 grams of carbohydrates. Eliminate the morning and evening snack. See snack recipes.

Day	Meal Item	Number of Calories/Carbs
Sun.		
Mon.		
Tues.		
Wed.		
Thurs.		
Fri.		
Sat.		

Lunch and Dinner:

Choose 1 lunch dish at 12 noon and 1 dinner dish at 6 p.m. containing less than 7 grams of carbs or choose a meal replacement drink unless you drank it earlier. See lunch and dinner recipes.

Day	Meal Item	Number of Calories/Carbs
Sun.		
Mon.		
Tues.		
Wed.		
Thurs.		
Fri.		
Sat.		

Metabolic Reset

After 12 to 16 weeks of dieting, you may take a break and eat 50 to 100 grams of carbs daily for 1 week to a month then resume the intermediate or advanced meal plan to re-start your ketogenic diet again. Most of the popular diets, recommend pushing the pause button on the diet to force the body to release the weight loss enzyme so smart beginners start losing more weight (Bradley 2018).

This break is necessary to reset your metabolism to lose more weight, if that's your goal. If you're ready to maintain your current weight, consume about 50 grams of carbs daily (Akers, 2017).

Be sure to track your weight so that it doesn't start creeping upward. If you're diabetic, be sure to track your glucose daily so that your numbers remain between 75 to 95 md/gl. Consult your doctor if you have any concerns during this reset period.

Energy & Exercise

When you enter nutritional ketosis, you receive a burst of energy. The energy level is phenomenal. That's why I think professional and amateur athletes prefer Keto to capture the energy level and control the number of carbs consumed.

To get to that energy level, you must enter nutritional or optimal ketosis. When your body starts running on ketones for energy, your energy level should go through the roof.

To get to nutritional or optimal ketosis faster, start an exercise routine (Mawer, 2018).

As previously mentioned, Start a regular exercise routine. Start slowly by taking little walks around the office or around the block. If you have a gym membership and are not applying it, start by going one day a week and working with one machine.

Don't start with the tread mill. Use one of the weight machines. Then increase your attendance to 2 days and use 2 machines. Stay off the tread mill until you are at least halfway to your big weight loss goal. Increase your attendance as you feel comfortable with and increase the usage of the machines.

It is always a good idea to ask a buddy to go with you to the gym. If you make an appointment to meet someone at the gym, you will be more likely to keep your date with the gym.

Fasting

The thought of fasting is daunting. Until you start practicing a fasting routine, the act itself keeps you guessing if you can hold out without eating for the length of time planned.

After you enter a fasting state, your body transitions into nutritional ketosis, turning your body into a fat-burning machine and diminishing your appetite. However, you must follow a few rules when you practice fasting (Clarke, 2019).

Fasting Rules

The following rules allows you to properly fast and stay healthy:

Consult with your doctor before fasting, especially if you have a medical condition that requires close monitoring.

Try 14-hour or 18-hour fasting to ease into not eating. Prepare and plan for fasting. Think about what you will drink and at what times during your fast. Don't rush into fasting on an impulse. Ensure your success and safety while fasting knowing that if you feel uncomfortable or overly hungry, stop the fasting period.

Listen to your body. If you feel faint or your stomach is upset, stop the fasting and consult your doctor or a healthcare professional.

Work the intermittent fasting practice around your life. If you have a big meeting at the office or if it's date night, skip this fasting period. You can focus on fasting later.

Stay hydrated. Drink lots of water or green or black tea. Don't drink any sugary drinks or juices. Those types of drinks make you crave carbs and may kick you out of ketosis.

Drink bone broth to get extra nutrients. Bone broth will make you feel full.

Take appropriate supplements like a multivitamin, MCT oil or electrolytes. MCT oil may curb your appetite and help you successfully fast. I practice the 18-hour fast during the week. I eat my last snack at 3 p.m., and then I drink a cup of coffee with MCT oil for dinner. I also drink my apple cider vinegar before bedtime, and I don't have another meal until the next morning at 8 a.m. I find it easy because I'm sleeping through most of the fasting hours. You may find fasting overnight easier and beneficial too.

Drink coffee wisely. Be careful not to load the coffee with cream or sugar. Sugar is a Keto no-no.

Eat normally. Do not binge eat. It's alright to stop the fasting period if you feel the need.

Stop the fasting period if you are under stress or at high stress times like during finals for college students, working long hours at the office, or meeting tough deadlines at home, work, or at school.

Exercise normally. Don't perform a strenuous workout routine. If you feel energized, take a walk or perform a light workout to attain nutritional or optimal ketosis. Be sure to test for ketosis.

Advantages

Several health advantages are associated with fasting such as:

- Lessens the risk of cancer

- Reduces the risk of heart disease

- Decreases triglyceride levels and blood pressure

- Boosts HDL (good) cholesterol levels

- Enhances autoimmune conditions

- Lowers blood sugar

- Improves metabolism

- Promotes weight loss

- Improves chronic inflammation

- Controls cravings

- Transitions the body toward ketosis

- Improves cognitive function

- Enhances lung health

- Diminishes inflammation in the large intestines

- Reduces bloating

Disadvantages

The disadvantages of fasting are as follows:

- Decreases energy

- Increases chance of dehydration

- Lowers level of electrolytes and minerals

- Increases chance of feeling dizzy or faint

- Lowers blood sugar levels

14-Hour Fasting Period

The 14-hour fasting period is the most normal fasting period if you skip dessert or not in the habit of raiding the refrigerator during the night. After you eat dinner at 6 p.m. (for example), you fast until tomorrow's breakfast at 8 a.m.

If you're a late-night eater, plan your fasting period around your routine to ensure a successful fast and to reap the rewards (Clarke, 2019).

18-Hour Fasting Period

The 18-hour fasting period is similar to the 14-hour but requires a little planning. For instance, you decide to begin after dinner at 6 p.m. Your next meal is tomorrow at 12 noon. It can be an easy time if you're not a big breakfast eater or if you plan ahead. Remember, you can drink water, coffee, protein shakes, green tea, vegetable smoothie drinks or broth during this time. Each drink helps curb your appetite, plus you'll be sleeping through the majority of this fasting period (Clarke, 2019).

Also remember, you're empowered to stop the fasting if you feel faint, dizzy or overly hungry. Be sure to take vitamins, supplements, or electrolytes to ensure a safe, successful fast.

24-Hour Fasting Period

The 24-hour fasting period is daunting and requires planning. You may want to write down what you'll drink and at what times. Once you write down your schedule, stick to it unless you need to stop the fasting period (Clarke, 2019).

Pick a 24-hour period when you're not busy or stressed. If you decide to fast from 6 p.m. to 6 p.m., write down your plan. For example, you eat dinner at 5:30 p.m. or so, and you drink 2 glasses of water between 6 p.m. to bedtime at 10 p.m. You sleep from 10 p.m. to 7 a.m., and then drink coffee or tea the next morning at 8 a.m. You continue to drink coffee, water, tea, or broth from 8 a.m. to 6 p.m. If you decide to take the MCT oil supplement at 8 a.m.

and 3 p.m., this supplement may help keep you from feeling hungry during what I call the lean times of the fasting period.

I've found that the 24-hour fasting period practice is better suited for once-a-week or once-a-month unless you know from testing that you are in nutritional or optimal ketosis.

Intermittent Fasting

Intermittent fasting is eating alternating days such as eating on Monday and Wednesday and fasting on Tuesday and Thursday. You don't have to fast the entire day. Smart beginners start with the 14-hour fast as described above whereas the more advanced seasoned dieters may perform the 18-hour or 24-hour fast. Ensure to follow the fasting rules (Clarke, 2019).

Fasting provides many health benefits. A smart beginner or a seasoned pro prepares and plans before jumping into the deep fasting pool. If you feel discomfort, dizziness, or faint, stop the fast. You may have to ease into the fasting practice to train your body and mind to accept the fasting condition.

Don't plan a fasting period during a special occasion such as during a work review, business trip, date night, high stressed outing, or strenuous exercise routine.

Consult your doctor or healthcare provider before starting a fasting routine and follow the fasting rules.

Stay hydrated by drinking plenty of water, broth, or herbal tea. Have fun while you turn your body into a fat burning machine.

STEP 5
JUMP THE DIETING HURDLES

Curing the Keto Flu

Stopping Food Cravings

Weight Loss Plateaus

Dining Out

Diet Cheating for Success

Curing the Keto Flu

As previously mentioned, the Keto Flu is what I called crossing the ketosis barrier. You may experience fatigue and headaches during this crossing phenomena.

The exact physiology is your body is having carb withdrawals and is adjusting from burning glucose to making and burning ketones as energy. Once you cross this barrier, the symptoms go away, and your body becomes a fat burning machine. It may take a couple of days to a couple of weeks for the Keto flu to pass.

Everyone is different; therefore, it's difficult to put an exact time on the recovery. However, the best part is your energy level goes through the roof when you're in nutritional or optimal ketosis.

To help you cope or avoid these symptoms, add the following remedies to your diet regimen (Hendon, 2020):

- Drink lots of water to avoid dehydration

- Drink bone broth for electrolytes and minerals

- Fast a meal or two. Refer to the chapter on Fasting

- Perform light exercises like walking or jogging

- Ensure you are getting enough salt or take multi-vitamin supplements to boost your electrolytes. Keto is actually a low-salt diet

- Eat some good carbs to boost your carb intake, but stay under 50 grams per day

- Take BHB and MCT oil supplements during this period to boost your ketone and good fat levels

Stopping the Food Cravings

Whenever I was on a diet, the biggest complaint I had was food cravings and feeling hungry. I asked doctors on occasion to prescribe me something to suppress my appetite and food cravings. They told me I didn't need an appetite suppressant and to eat more fiber. Fiber diminishes hunger. However, doctors could have prescribed medicine to suppress my hunger, but these drugs are a temporary fix to an overlying problem.

One of the best virtues of the Keto diet is that it suppresses appetite and food cravings (Ciccarelli, 2018).

However, before my Keto diet and when I was dieting and fasting between meals or on a daily routine, I suffered because of uncontrollable cravings. These cravings were mostly everything I could not eat while on the diet. Therefore, the diet became short lived because the cravings became so great that I had to surrender. Eventually, I caved to the cravings. If you are like me, you have experienced this phenomenon too.

After I started my Keto diet, at around the 10th day and once my body started producing ketones as energy, all my appetite and food cravings stopped. Even when I fasted for 12 to 24 hours, I could fast with ease because I didn't feel hungry.

If you need to re-read how the Keto diet works with your digestive enzymes, refer to the chapter on How Weight Loss Works for the nuts and bolts about enzymes and how they work to promote weight loss.

If you feel hungry and need a snack, eat a boiled egg, two cherry tomatoes with a half stick of celery or a fat bomb (see recipes).

Several nutritional and supplement companies produce Keto supplements to help keep you in ketosis and to suppress the phenomenon of feeling hungry. See Keto Supplements for more information. Be careful to pick supplements containing no fillers or hiding high net carbs.

Weight Loss Plateaus

One strange diet phenomenon is weight loss plateaus. You will be making huge progress losing 2 to 4 pounds at a time then "pow." You can't get the scale to move off a particular number. It can last a few days to a few months. It's frustrating.

After 8 weeks on the diet, I found myself on a diet plateau. I first tried to fast my way off it. Then I ate about 2200 calories in one day with about 60 grams of net carbs. The next morning, to my surprise, the scale showed I lost 1.5 pounds. I had shocked my body off the plateau and started losing weight again.

I wanted to learn more about plateaus, so I did some research. I found the following causes and solutions to this mysterious phenomenon (Keto diet weight loss plateau: what to consider and how to break it, 2018):

Causes

- Consuming too many carbs

- Kicking yourself out of ketosis

- Eating too many calories

- Ingesting the wrong types of foods

- Not eating real whole foods

- Eating too many nuts

- Not fasting, especially intermittent fasting

- Approaching goal weight

- Not getting enough sleep or poor sleep habits

- Becoming stressed out

- Dealing with thyroid and adrenal issues

Solutions

- Consume less than 30 carbs daily

- Test ketosis level

- Eat less than 800 calories, once or twice a week

- Follow the chapter on What Foods to Eat and What Foods to Avoid

- Eat fewer nuts; see chapter on What Foods to Minimize

- Practice intermittent or 24-hour fasting

- Get plenty of sleep (at least 8 hours if possible)

- Re-analyze or rethink your stress situation

- See your doctor or healthcare provider about thyroid or adrenal issues

Dining Out

If you stocked your pantry with Keto friendly foods, eating at home becomes less stressful because you have rid your pantry of the tempting foods. If you pack your lunch for work and only eat what you take to work, eating at the workplace becomes less of an ordeal.

If your co-workers insist that you go to lunch with them, tell them you are on Keto. They will back down on insisting, or they will become inquisitive. If they become inquisitive, you can point them to the information you learned.

However, dining out becomes a different type of a struggle. My wife and I used to enjoy dining out once a week, and we enjoyed takeout from restaurants two to three times a week. After starting Keto, we dined out once a month for special occasions like birthdays or anniversaries.

With the knowledge of Keto, eating out becomes fun again because you know What Foods to Eat.

- Choose leafy vegetables over potatoes, corn, or beans

- Choose meat containing less calories if you track calories and carbs like white fish, cod, or salmon

- Don't choose an appetizer because most are made on some type of bread

- Don't eat rolls, biscuits, or bread

- Skip dessert if possible

- Don't drink a mixed alcoholic drink or soda (or diet soda)

Diet Cheating for Success

You need to be strict with yourself while on the Keto diet, restricting and counting carbs and counting calories. After you've been on the diet for about two months, the diet fascination starts to become stale. It's OK to take a break for physiological and psychological reasons. However, if you choose not to take a break, that's OK too.

Sometimes, especially if you are on a diet plateau, your body needs a shock of eating higher calories or higher carbs while you're taking a break for a day.

I cheated on my diet with one day here and another day there. As I previously stated, after 8 weeks on the diet, I found myself on a diet plateau. I first tried to fast my way off of it. Then I ate about 2200 calories with about 60 grams of net carbs. That did the trick. To my surprise, the scale showed I lost 1.5 pounds. Then I got back with the rigors of the diet to continue my success.

My first real test came when I went out of town to my wife's niece's wedding. The wedding happened the day after the Thanksgiving holidays.

The festivities regarding the wedding and the holidays would normally put a strain on my diet. I thought if I stray from the diet, the meal must be close to being Keto friendly, being meat of some type, vegetables with little or no bread.

To start off each day, the hotel offered a full breakfast with eggs, bacon, sausage, pancakes, donuts, coffee, cereal, bagels, and so on. Who could pass up a breakfast like that?

In the evening of the rehearsal dinner and then the wedding reception, with the mindset of being on vacation and being in the atmosphere or the cuisine of the festivities, who could pass up the wonderful meals and trappings? Therefore, I participated and ate the meals with the trimmings and dessert that I could muster.

I took travel packages of MCT oil and BHB exogenesis supplements to help me stay in ketosis. Depending on how many carbs I consumed, these supplements were outstanding. I did not feel fatigued or have a headache. However, if you have the option, I recommend staying strict with Keto diet for at least two months. I had been on Keto for three months.

However, my wife and I came away unscathed. We did not gain or lose any weight during that trip. I don't recommend cheating on your diet if you can stay true to the diet and yourself. I know that circumstances and feelings cause you to make decisions outside of the box. Therefore, if you do have to make these decisions, choose foods to help keep you in ketosis, and if necessary, take a Keto supplement to make your cheating successful.

If you do stray away to keep your sanity, it's OK to take a break for a day or a week to gain newfound commitment. Keep in mind if you get kicked out of ketosis, you may cross the ketosis barrier, only to experience the Keto flu again.

However, when you do take a break, revisit my chapter Dining Out to make wiser diet choices while taking a break. Don't start eating a high carb diet just because you want or desire it. Remember too, eating in moderation is better than eating everything in sight or at will.

If you stray away from your Keto diet, don't stay away too long, especially if you have a health condition that feeds on carbs like diabetes, cancer, Alzheimer's, and so on. You must starve these diseases of their carbs to keep control and/or to conquer them (Kossoff, 2017).

RECIPES

Breakfast Recipes

Baked Avocado with Egg

Boiled Eggs

No Crust Breakfast Ham and Cheese Quiche

Lunch and Dinner Recipes

Egg Roll Bowl Unwrapped

Slow Cooker Chicken Tortilla Soup

Spinach and Cilantro Stuffed Chicken Breast

Slow Cooker Jambalaya

Old Fashioned Southern Style Meatloaf

Salmon Croquette with Dill Garlic Dip

Snack Recipes

Peanut Butter & Chocolate Fat Bomb

Pepperoni Pizza Mushroom Poppers

Deviled Salmon Eggs

Cooking Conversions

Dry/Weight Measurements

Liquid or Volume Measurements

Conversions for Baking Ingredients

Oven Temperatures

Breakfast Recipes

Baked Avocado with Egg

This meal contains only 6 ingredients. It's easy to assemble. To enhance this dish, add crispy bacon.

Course: Breakfast

Prep Time: 5 to 10 minutes

Cook Time: 15 to 20 minutes

Total Time: 20 to 30 minutes

Ingredients (alphabetized)

Avocados – 3, cut in half and remove seed

Cheese – 1 tablespoon of Mexican blend of Sharp Cheddar, Colby, and Monterrey Jack, shredded

Eggs – 6 medium or small

Pepper – 1 pinch, to taste

Salsa – (Optional), to taste

Salt – 1 pinch, to taste

Directions

1. Preheat oven to 375 degrees Fahrenheit. Lightly oil baking sheet or coat with nonstick spray.

2. Scoop, with a spoon, about 2 tablespoons of avocado flesh as needed, creating a small well in the center of each avocado.

3. Gently crack 1 egg, and slide it into the avocado well, keeping the yolk intact.

4. Repeat with remaining eggs. Season each with salt and pepper.

5. Place into oven and bake until the egg whites are set but the yolks are still runny, about 15 to 18 minutes. If you like the yolks firm, then leave in oven till yolks are firm. Keep an eye on the eggs so that they don't get overcooked.

6. Serve immediately, garnish with cheese and salsa, to taste if desired.

Cooking Tips

Avocados should be ripe. If the avocados are too green or too brown, the taste of the avocado will overpower the eggs.

Small eggs are easier to handle and may not create such a mesh in the oven if it overflows. Plus, the egg white may become crispy which is always an added bonus.

Nutritional Facts

Serving: 1 serving

Calories: 232

Fat: 19.7 g

Sodium: 69.8 mg

Total Carbs: 9.5 g

Net Carbs: 2.7 g

Fiber: 6.8 g

Sugar: 1.1 g

Protein: 7.9 g

Boiled Eggs

Course: Breakfast

Prep Time: 1 minutes

Cook Time: 7 to 9 minutes

Total Time: 17 to 23 minutes

Ingredients (alphabetized)

Cold Water

Eggs – 6 large, cold from refrigerator

Ice

Salt or Baking Soda – 1 teaspoon (depending on the age of the eggs)

Directions

1. Place eggs in a large saucepan. Cover eggs with cool water by 1 inch. Add salt or baking soda to pan.

2. Cover the pan with a lid and bring water to a rolling boil over high heat. When water is boiling, set time for desired time as follows in step 3.

3. Boil for 6 to 7 minutes over medium-high heat for perfect hard-boiled eggs.

4. Take eggs out of hot water with slotted spoon and put in bowl. Place ice in bowl to stop the eggs' cooking process. After eggs have cooled (about 10 to 15 minutes), crack, peel, and serve.

Cooking Tips

Boil for 4 to 5 minutes for soft-boiled eggs. Boil for 7 to 9 minutes for harder boiled eggs.

Adding salt to the water raises the boiling point of the water.

The salt also seals the eggshell if a crack or leak occurs and keeps the egg yolks from running all over the sauce pan by helping the egg coagulate if the eggs crack while boiling. The salt also makes the eggs easier to peel. It's not fool-proof because some eggs can be a bad or tough-to-peel egg.

Adding baking soda to the cooking water increases the boiling point too. Be careful that your boiling water don't overflow while reaching its boiling point. However, if the eggs are older, they are more alkaline, and by adding baking soda, the soda will increase the alkalinity, making the eggs easier to peel.

It's ok to add both salt and baking soda. Both ingredients react the same with the water and the eggs. By adding both to the water may be overkill or wasteful. I am guilty of putting both in the water, but I tend to think my eggs' shells are tender when peeling.

Nutritional Facts

Serving: 1 Hard-Boiled Egg

Calories: 77.5

Fat: 5.3 g

Sodium: 62 mg

Total Carbs: 0.6 g

Net Carbs: 0.6 g

Fiber: 0 g

Sugar: 0.6 g

Protein: 6.3 g

No Crust Breakfast Ham and Cheese Quiche

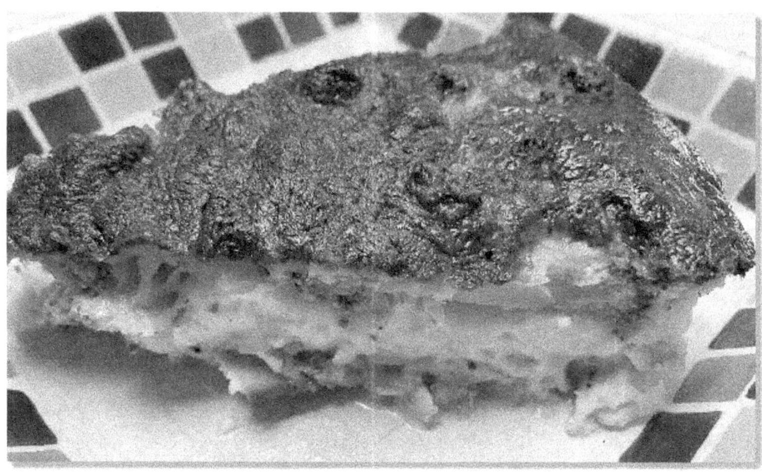

This dish is a great meal to make ahead of time and store in the refrigerator for up to 5 days or in the freezer for up to 1 month.

Course: Breakfast

Prep Time: 10 to 15 minutes

Cook Time: 47 to 55 minutes

Total Time: 57 to 70 minutes

Ingredients (alphabetized)

Baby Broccoli Florets – 2 cups

Butter – 1 tablespoon

Cheese – 8 ounces of Mexican blend of Sharp Cheddar, Colby, and Monterrey Jack, shredded

Eggs – 6 large

Ham – 8 ounces, cubed

Heavy Cream – 1 cup

Yellow Onion – ½ cup, diced

Directions

1. Preheat oven to 375 degrees Fahrenheit.

2. Melt butter, over medium heat in a skillet, and add onions and ham. Sauté for 5 to 7 minutes until onions are translucent.

3. Place baby broccoli florets in a microwave-safe bowl and add 2 tablespoons of water. Microwave for 2 to 3 minutes until broccoli is lightly steamed and tender.

4. In a bowl, add eggs and heavy cream. Whisk together.

5. Place ham, onions, broccoli, and cheese in a greased 9-inch pie plate or quiche pan.

6. Pour the egg mixture over the meat and vegetables.

7. Place in the oven and bake for 35 to 40 minutes or until the quiche center is firm and doesn't shake.

8. Remove and let stand (cool) for about 5 minutes before cutting and serving.

Cooking Tips

Add garlic and green peppers while sautéing the onions to enhance the flavor.

Bake this dish and let cool for 20 minutes, and then wrap with a polyethylene plastic such as Saran Wrap or in a freezer safe container and freeze for up to 1 month.

To eat from the freezer, unwrap the quiche from the polyethylene plastic and place in the microwave for 2 to 5 minutes (depending on your microwave and power setting) and enjoy.

Nutritional Facts

Serving: 1 slice

Calories: 319

Fat: 26 g

Sodium: 619 mg

Total Carbs: 5 g

Net Carbs: 4 g

Fiber: 1 g

Sugar: 2 g

Protein: 17 g

Lunch and Dinner Recipes

Egg Roll Bowl Unwrapped

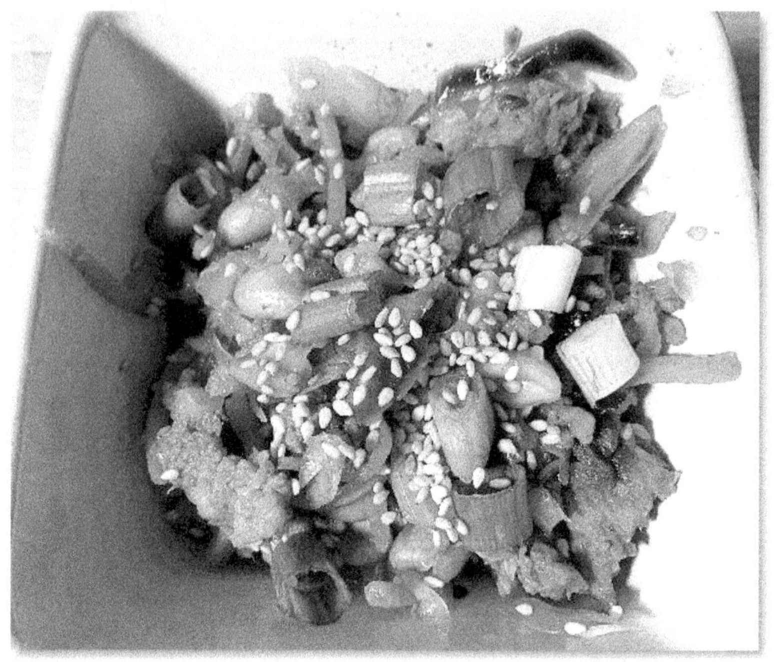

Course: Lunch or Dinner

Prep Time: 10 minutes

Cook Time: 15 minutes

Total Time: 25 minutes

Ingredients (alphabetized)

Beef – ½ pound ground

Beef Bone Broth – 1/3 cup

Cabbage – 14 ounces, shredded or broccoli coleslaw

Carrot – 1 medium, shredded

Garlic – 1 teaspoon minced, and 5 cloves sliced

Ginger – 1 teaspoon minced

Green onions – 2 or 3, chopped

Hoisin sauce – 1 tablespoon, to taste

Onion – 1 small, diced (chopped)

Pepper – to taste

Pork – ½ pound ground

Rice vinegar – 2 teaspoons

Salt – to taste

Sesame oil – 1 tablespoon

Sesame seeds – 2 teaspoons

Soy Sauce – ¼ cup low sodium

Sriracha – 1 tablespoon

Directions

1. Heat large skillet over medium heat. Add olive oil and ground beef and pork. Cook until browned and cooked through.

2. Add onions, garlic, and ginger to skillet. Stir well, and cook until softened and translucent, about 5 minutes.

3. Make sesame oil mixture by combining sesame oil, soy sauce, Sriracha, hoisin sauce, and rice vinegar in a measuring cup, and stir to combine.

4. Add cabbage and carrot and broth. Stir to coat. Add sesame oil mixture to skillet. Stir to coat.

5. Cook, stirring regularly for 5 minutes until softened. Cover skillet with lid so that the cabbage will reduce. Keep covered

for 3 to 5 minutes depending on how soft you want the cabbage.

6. Garnish with green onions and sesame seeds.

Nutritional Facts

Serving: 1

Yield: 6

Calories: 380

Fat: 24 g

Total Carbs: 5 g

Net Carbs: 3 g

Fiber: 2 g

Protein: 26 g

Slow Cooker Chicken Tortilla Soup

Course: Lunch or Dinner

Prep Time: 10 minutes

Cook Time: 4 hours

Total Time: 4 hours 10 minutes

Ingredients (alphabetized)

Adobo Seasoning – 2 teaspoons

Butter – 2 tablespoons

Chicken Bone Broth – 2 cups

Chicken Breast – 1 pound, boneless and skinless

Chicken Thighs – 1 pound, boneless and skinless

Colby or Colby Jack Cheese – 8 ounces, shredded

Heavy Cream – ¼ cup

Pepper Jack Cheese – 8 ounces, shredded

Salsa – 1 cup, low-carb

Salt – 1 teaspoon

Whole Wheat Tortillas – 3, low-carb

Xanthan Gum or Corn Starch – 1 tablespoon (optional)

Directions

1. Place chicken, cream, salsa, adobo seasoning and salt in the slow cooker pot. Cook on low for 4 hours or until chicken is completely cooked.

2. Take chicken out of the slow cooker and shred it, and then add the chicken back into the slow cooker pot.

3. Pour in the broth and half of each of the cheeses.

4. Add 1 teaspoon of xanthan gum to thicken soup (optional).

5. Cook on low for one more hour or until cheese is melted.

6. Make the tortilla strips while soup is cooking. Dredge through butter and place on a pan and bake on 350 degrees for 10 to 15 minutes. Do not burn.

7. Serve the soup with the remaining shredded cheeses and tortilla strips.

Nutritional Facts

Serving: 1

Calories: 619

Fat: 48 g

Sodium: X mg

Total Carbs: 7 g

Net Carbs: 6 g

Fiber: 1 g

Sugar: 4 g

Protein: 40 g

Spinach and Cilantro Stuffed Chicken Breast

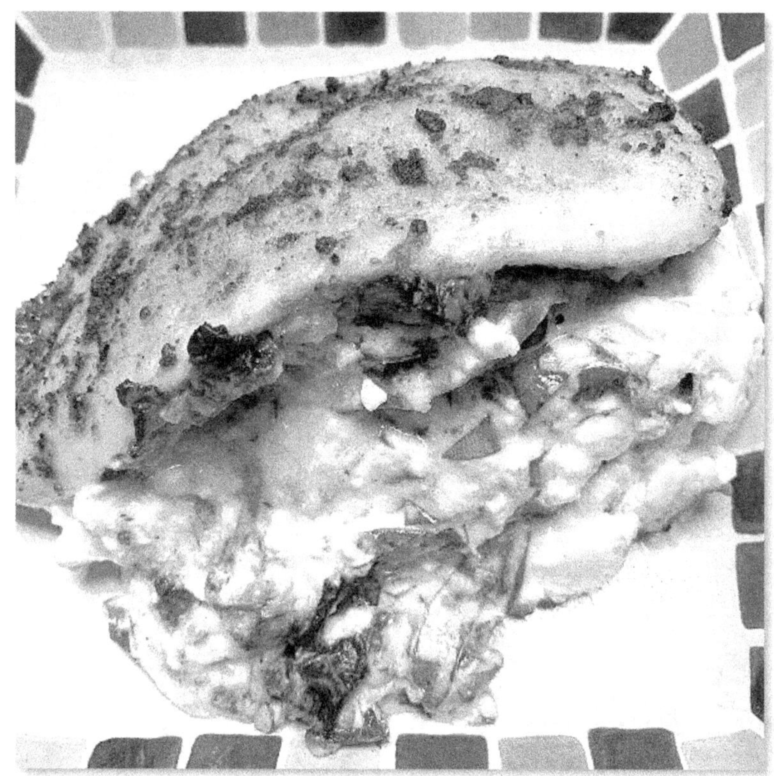

Course: Lunch or Dinner

Prep Time: 10 minutes

Cook Time: 25 minutes

Total Time: 35 minutes

Ingredients (alphabetized)

Chicken Breast – 4, boneless and skinless

Chili Powder – ¼ teaspoon

Cilantro – 1/8 cup, chopped fresh, to taste (optional)

Cream Cheese – 4 ounces, softened

Dill Seasoning – 1 teaspoon

Garlic – 2 cloves, minced

Garlic Powder – ¼ teaspoon

Mayonnaise – 2 tablespoons

Olive Oil – 1 tablespoon

Onion Powder – ¼ teaspoon

Parmesan Cheese – ¼ cup, grated

Salt – 1 teaspoon, divided

Smoked Paprika – 1 teaspoon

Spinach – 1-1/2 cups chopped, fresh

Directions

1. Preheat oven to 375 degrees Fahrenheit.

2. Place the chicken breast on a cutting board. Use a sharp knife to cut a pocket into the side of each chicken breast.

3. Drizzle olive oil on each chicken breast and set aside.

4. Add the smoked paprika, ½ teaspoon salt, garlic powder, onion powder, dill seasoning, and chili powder to a small bowl and stir to combine. Sprinkle evenly over both sides of the chicken breast.

5. Add cream cheese, Parmesan, mayonnaise, spinach, cilantro, garlic and the other ½ teaspoon of salt to a small mixing bowl and stir well to combine.

6. Spoon the spinach and cilantro mixture into each chicken breast (pocket) evenly. Pack the mixture so that none of the cream cheese is exposed.

7. Place chicken breast in a 9x13 inch baking dish.

8. Bake, uncovered for 25 minutes or until the chicken's internal temperature reaches 165 degrees Fahrenheit (75 degrees Celsius).

Cooking Tips

Use the dry ingredients as a rub to coat the chicken prior to baking.

Cilantro tends to be overpowering. Use less cilantro than recommended if you are sensitive or dislike the taste. It is ok to use only spinach without the cilantro too.

When the chicken's internal temperature reaches 165 degrees Fahrenheit (75 degrees Celsius), the chicken is cooked through and the juices should run clear.

If you don't like the taste of baked garlic, you can use 1 teaspoon of minced garlic or omit it completely.

Nutritional Facts

Serving: 1 chicken breast

Calories: 407

Fat: 24 g

Sodium: 873 mg

Total Carbs: 3 g

Net Carbs: 2 g

Fiber: 1 g

Protein: 41 g

Slow Cooker Jambalaya with Chicken, Shrimp & Sausage

Make this Keto-friendly New Orleans classic style dish with cauliflower rice.

Course: Lunch or Dinner

Prep Time: 30 minutes

Cook Time: 4 hours

Total Time: 4 hours and 30 minutes

Ingredients (alphabetized)

Andouille Sausage – 4 links, halved lengthwise and sliced

Cajun Seasoning, Salt Free – 2 tablespoons

Cauliflower Rice – One (16-ounce) bag

Celery – 2 stalks, chopped

Chicken Breast – 2 halves, boneless and skinless

Chicken Thighs – 4, boneless and skinless

Garlic – 4 cloves, minced or chopped

Hot Sauce – ½ teaspoon or to taste

Olive Oil – 4 tablespoons, divided

Onion – 1 large, finely chopped

Parsley, Fresh – ¼ cup, chopped, divided

Pepper – ½ teaspoon

Red Bell Pepper – 1, chopped

Salt – ½ teaspoon

Smoked Paprika – 1 tablespoon

Shrimp– 8 ounces, large peeled and deveined

Tomatoes, Petite Diced – 1 (15-ounce) can, undrained

Directions

1. Place cauliflower rice on bottom of slow cooker. Heat slow cooker pot on low to medium while you prepare the chicken, sausage, and shrimp.

2. Heat 2 to 3 tablespoons of olive oil in large nonstick skillet. When skillet is hot, brown chicken in skillet for 3 to 6 minutes. Do not cook the chicken completely. The slow cooker will finish the cooking.

3. Place chicken, Cajun seasoning, salt and pepper in the slow cooker pot.

4. Add onion, celery, red bell pepper, garlic, and smoked paprika, hot sauce, tomatoes, and 1/8 cup of parsley to slow cooker.

5. Cook on low for 4 hours or until chicken is completely cooked.

6. Add Andouille sausage and shrimp and cook on low for the last hour. You may need to adjust the cooking time for the sausage and shrimp so that it is not overcooked.

7. After chicken is cooked through, cut chicken into 1/2-inch pieces.

8. Adjust seasonings, to taste, and serve. Garnish with remaining parsley.

Cooking Tips

Do not cook the chicken completely when browning it in skillet.

You may need to adjust the cooking time for the sausage and shrimp so that it is not overcooked.

Nutritional Facts

Serving: 1 cup

Yield: 8 to 12

Calories: 260

Fat: 15 g

Sodium: 1460 mg

Total Carbs: 11 g

Net Carbs: 6.5 g

Fiber: 4.5 g

Sugar: 5 g

Protein: 21.5 g

Old Fashioned Southern Style Meatloaf

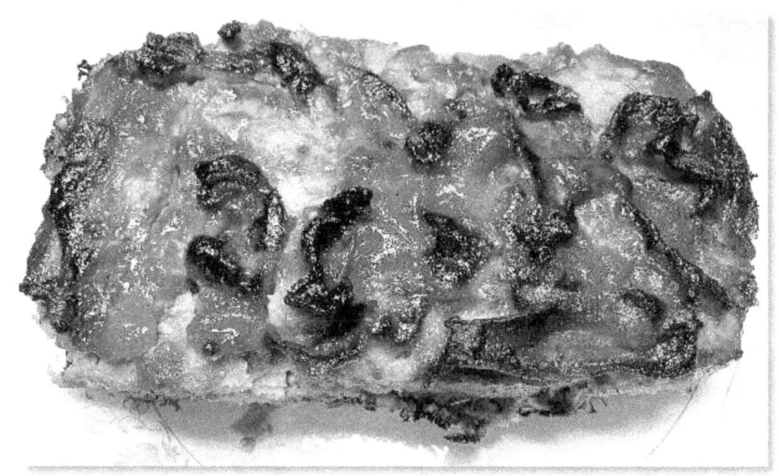

Course: Lunch or Dinner

Prep Time: 10 minutes

Cook Time: 45 minutes

Total Time: 55 minutes

Ingredients (alphabetized)

Almond Flour – ¼ cup

Bacon – 3 to 4 slices, (Applewood)

Basil, 1 teaspoon

Beef, Ground – ½ pound

Bell Pepper, Green – 1

Cheddar, Shredded – ½ cup

Eggs – 2 large

Garlic – 1 clove, minced (1 teaspoon)

Garlic Salt – ¼ teaspoon

Hot sauce – 1 teaspoon, to taste

Italian Salad Dressing – 1 tablespoon

Italian Seasoning, 1 teaspoon

Ketchup, Unsweetened – 3 tablespoons (Primal Kitchen)

Onion – ½ onion

Onion Powder – ½ teaspoon

Parmesan Cheese, Powdered – ¼ cup

Pepper, Black – 1 teaspoon

Pork, Ground – ½ pound

Salt – 1 teaspoon

Worcestershire Sauce – 1 tablespoon

Directions

1. Preheat oven to 375 degrees Fahrenheit (190 degrees Celsius).

2. Chop green bell pepper, onion, and mince garlic.

3. Add to a large bowl with ground beef, ground pork, eggs, almond flour, cheddar, Parmesan cheese, Worcestershire sauce, basil, garlic salt, onion powder, Italian seasoning, salt, and pepper. Combine ingredients with your hands.

4. Shape mixture into a loaf and place in a 9x13 baking dish or meatloaf pan.

5. Cut bacon slices in thirds and drape of meatloaf.

6. Bake for 25 minutes.

7. Whisk together the ketchup, hot sauce, and Italian dressing. Spoon half of the mixture over the meatloaf.

8. Increase heat to 425 degrees Fahrenheit (220 degrees Celsius) and bake an additional 10 minutes then spread the remaining sauce over the meatloaf.

9. Continue baking for 10 to 15 minutes or until the internal temperature reaches 160 degrees Fahrenheit (71 degrees Celsius).

10. Let meatloaf rest for 5 minutes before removing from dish or pan and slicing. Garnish with parsley, serve, and enjoy.

Nutritional Facts

Nutritional facts are generated by Sparkpeople.com recipe nutrition calculator. Facts may vary.

Serving: 1 slice

Yield: 6 slices

Calories: 377.3

Fat: 29.1 g

Saturated Fat 10.8 g

Polyunsaturated Fat 2.3 g

Monounsaturated Fat 10.1 g

Cholesterol 134.6 mg

Sodium: 803.1 mg

Potassium 261.3 mg

Total Carbs: 7.8 g

Net Carbs: 6.6 g

Fiber: 1.2 g

Protein: 21 g

Salmon Croquette with Dill Garlic Dip

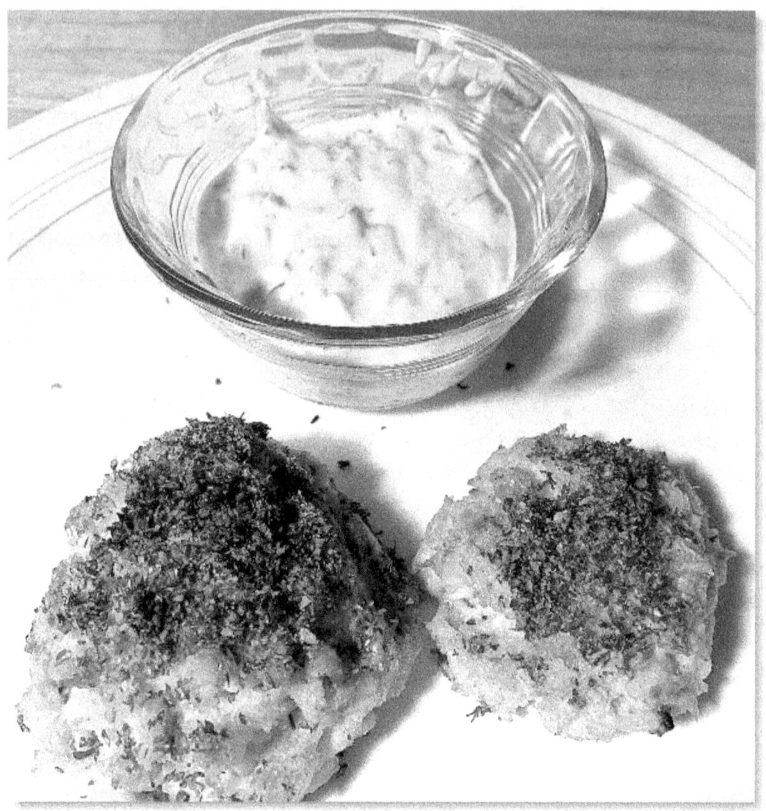

Course: Lunch or Dinner

Prep Time: 15 minutes

Cook Time: 15 minutes

Total Time: 30 minutes

Ingredients

Salmon Croquette (alphabetized)

Almond Flour – ½ cup

Egg – 1 large

Mayonnaise – 2 tablespoons

Olive oil – 2 tablespoons

Pepper – ½ teaspoon, black

Salmon – 6 ounce can, drained

Salt – 3/4 teaspoon

Thyme – ¼ teaspoon, ground

Dill – ½ teaspoon, finely chopped (optional)

Dill Garlic Dip

Sour Cream – ½ cup

Dill – 1 tablespoon, fresh finely chopped

Garlic – 4 cloves, minced

Red Pepper Flakes – ¼ teaspoon

Directions

1. Combine dill garlic dip ingredients: sour cream, dill, minced garlic, red pepper flakes, ¼ teaspoon of salt, and ¼ teaspoon of pepper, and stir until well mixed. Cover and refrigerate.

2. Drain canned salmon and discard any bones and skin. Pat salmon meat dry with paper towels. Use a digital food scale to measure out 6 ounces of salmon to use for this recipe if can failed to list the drained weight or if you removed a lot of bones and skin.

3. Add salmon croquette ingredients: salmon, almond flour, mayonnaise, egg, ½ teaspoon of salt, thyme, and ¼ teaspoon of black pepper in a large mixing bowl, and stir until well mixed. Break apart any large chunks of salmon. Divide the mixture

into 5 equal sized balls and use a spatula to flatten them into 2 to 3-inch patties or roll into a tight ball.

4. Heat olive oil in a large skillet (big enough to accommodate 5 patties without crowding) over a medium heat until hot.

5. Use spatula to carefully lower patties, one at a time, evenly spaced into the hot oil. Tilt the skillet to ensure good oil coverage around all patties.

6. Fry until the patties or ball are browned and crispy on the bottom, about 5 to 6 minutes. Flip the patties and repeat for the other side, about 3 to 4 minutes. Take the patties from the skillet and place on a paper towel to drain.

7. Place salmon patties on serving plates. Garnish (optional) with fresh dill on top of each salmon patty or ball. Take dill garlic dip from refrigerator and spoon a dollop of dip on top of each patty. Spoon the remainder of the dip on the side. Serve salmon croquettes while hot and crispy.

Cooking Tips

Press the salmon flat into patties on a nonstick surface with parchment paper or roll into round ball if preferred. Sprinkle almond flour on the parchment paper to provide enough traction so that the patties don't stick to the paper.

Garnish salmon croquettes with dill or flax seed (optional).

Nutritional Facts

Serving: 1 croquette
Calories: 290
Fat: 26 g
Sodium: 420 mg
Total Carbs: 3.5 g

Net Carbs: 2 g
Fiber: 1.5 g
Sugar: 1.5 g
Protein: 11 g

Snack Recipes

Peanut Butter & Chocolate Fat Bomb

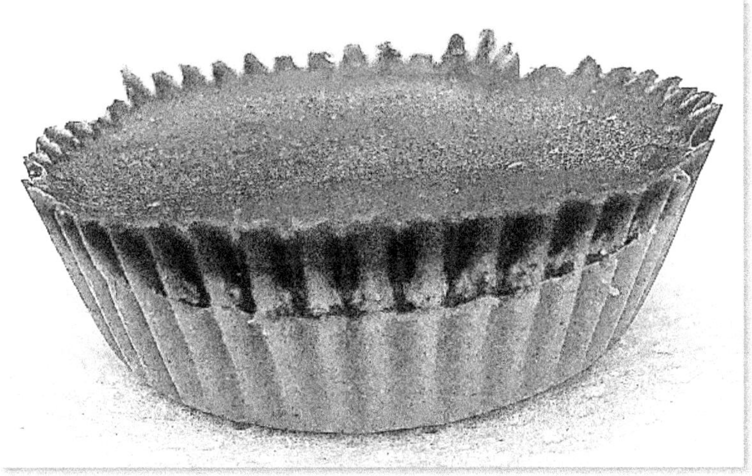

This bomb satisfies your sweet tooth. This snack is my all-time favorite. It tastes just like the famous peanut butter cup candy we enjoyed as a kid. However, this snack is better for you because of the coconut (good) fat.

Course: Snack

Prep Time: 5 minutes

Chill Time: 1 hour 30 minutes

Total Time: 5 minutes

Ingredients (alphabetized)

Peanut Butter Bottom Portion

Coconut Butter – ¼ cup, softened

Coconut Flour – 2 tablespoons

Coconut Oil – ¼ cup, softened

Peanut Butter – ¾ cup

Pecans – ¼ cup, chopped (optional)

Stevia – liquid, 4 drops

Vanilla Extract – ¼ teaspoon

Chocolate Top Portion

Cocoa Powder – 2 to 4 tbsp

Coconut Butter – 4 tbsp, softened

Coconut Flour – 2 tablespoons

Stevia – liquid, 2 drops

Directions

1. In a small microwave safe bowl, soften the coconut and peanut butter in the microwave (about 15 to 30 seconds on high).

2. Combine the melted coconut and peanut butter, salt, vanilla extract, coconut flour, and liquid stevia. Beat or whisk until well combined.

3. Place paper muffin cups in muffin pan.

4. Spoon 3 tablespoons of peanut butter mixture into paper muffin cups.

5. Repeat until all paper muffin cups are filled.

6. Chill in refrigerator freezer for 1 hour.

7. In a small microwave safe bowl, soften the coconut butter and coconut oil in microwave (about 15 seconds on high).

8. Add cocoa powder and liquid stevia to coconut butter and coconut oil to make chocolate top portion.

9. Spoon 1 to 1-1/2 tablespoons or pour chocolate top portion on top of the peanut butter bottom portion. Ensure that the bottom is firm.

10. Chill in refrigerator freezer for 30 minutes to 1 hour before serving.

Cooking Tips

If storing for lunches, place the bombs in a food storage container and refrigerate till needed.

The coconut flour is used for thickening. If the coconut oil and butter is thickening without the flour, you may omit it.

The bombs also can be stored up to 3 months in the freezer.

Nutritional Facts

Serving: 1

Yield: 6 to 12

Calories: 194

Fat: 24 g

Sodium: 30 mg

Total Carbs: 6 g

Net Carbs: 1 g

Fiber: 5 g

Sugar: 1 g

Protein: 5 g

Pepperoni Pizza Mushroom Poppers

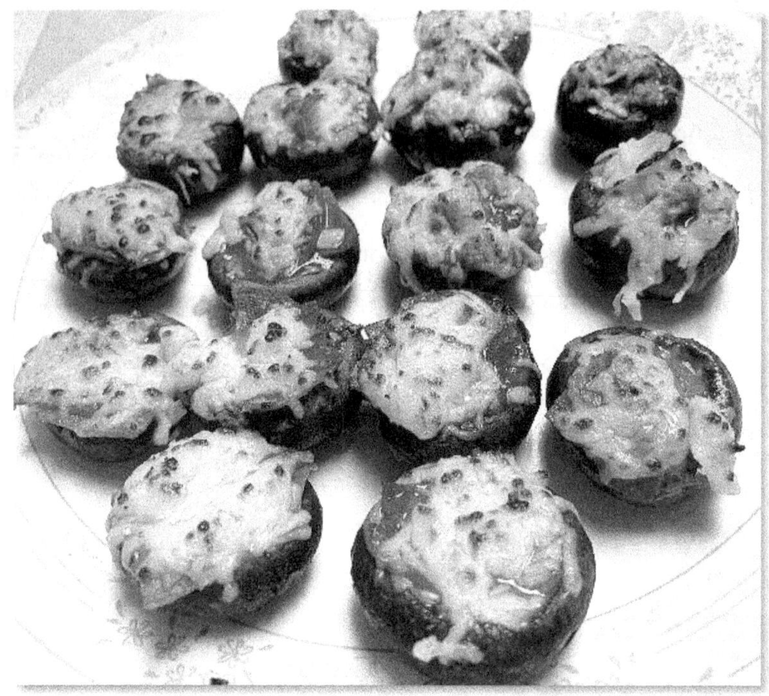

These Pizza Mushroom Poppers taste great. It's just like eating a pepperoni mushroom pizza without a huge amount of carbs. This snack is great for tailgating parties.

Course: Snack

Prep Time: 10 minutes

Cook Time: 15 minutes

Total Time: 25 minutes

Ingredients (alphabetized)

8-ounce package of mushrooms (white or baby bella)

1 tbsp olive oil

1/4 cup pizza sauce

8 pieces of turkey or regular pepperoni

1/2 cup of mozzarella cheese (shredded)

2 tbsp of diced jalapeno peppers (optional)

Directions

1. Preheat oven to 400 degrees F.

2. Brush dirt from mushrooms with a damp cloth. Do not rinse mushroom under faucet.

3. Pop stems and scoop membranes out with spoon.

4. Brush mushrooms outsides with olive oil.

5. Bake mushrooms 5 to 10 minutes till tender but firm.

6. Remove mushrooms from oven.

7. Change the setting to broil.

8. Fill each mushroom cavity with pizza sauce.

9. Top sauce with pepperoni and mozzarella cheese.

10. Return mushroom to oven and broil for about 2 minutes or until the cheese is melted.

Cooking Tips

Mushrooms contain a lot of water. If your mushrooms start accumulating water in the pan, pull them out of oven and drain.

Be careful handling the HOT pan. Suffering a second- or third-degree burn is no fun. I still have my scar from my grilling expedition.

Keep a close eye on the mushrooms. The broil settings on most ovens tend to burn if overlooked.

Nutritional Facts

Nutritional facts are generated by Sparkpeople.com recipe nutrition calculator. Facts may vary.

Serving: 1 Popper

Yield: 10

Calories: 54.8

Fat: 4.5 g

Saturated Fat: 1.6 g

Polyunsaturated Fat: 0.3 g

Monounsaturated Fat: 2.2 g

Sodium: 148.2 mg

Potassium: 51.3 mg

Total Carbs: 1.3 g

Net Carbs: 1 g

Fiber: 0.3 g

Sugar: 0.5 g

Protein: 2.6 g

Deviled Salmon Eggs

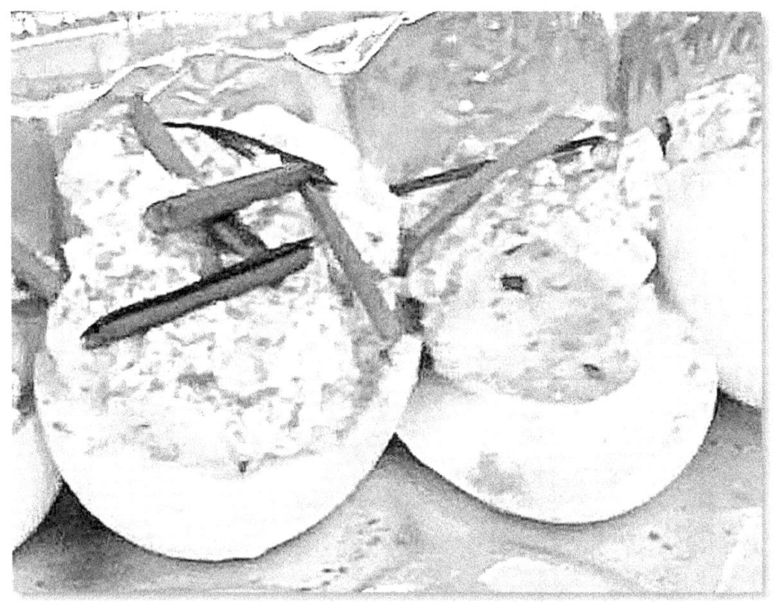

This snack dish is perfect for the holidays or office special occasions. Surprise your co-workers with a healthy tasty snack.

Course: Snack

Prep Time: 10 minutes

Cook Time: 15 minutes

Total Time: 25 minutes

Ingredients (alphabetized)

Chives, Fresh – 1 tablespoon, minced

Cream Cheese – 4 ounces, softened

Dill – 1 teaspoon

Eggs – 6, large

Horseradish – 1 teaspoon

Lemon Juice, Fresh – 1 tablespoon

Mayonnaise – 1 tablespoon

Mustard, Spicy Brown – 1 teaspoon

Paprika, Smoked – ¼ teaspoon or shaker

Pepper, Black – ¼ teaspoon

Salmon, Smoked – 2.5-ounce package

Salt – ¼ teaspoon

Sour Cream – 1 tablespoon

Directions

1. Make hard boiled eggs.

2. Peel eggs, and cut each egg in half lengthwise, and remove the egg yolks to a bowl.

3. Add cream cheese, sour cream, lemon juice, chives, mayonnaise, mustard, horseradish, dill, salmon, salt, and pepper to the yolk bowl. Stir well and taste the mixture to ensure it's seasoned to your taste.

4. Spoon the mixture into each of the egg halves.

5. Garnish eggs with smoked paprika and chives. Keep chilled in the refrigerator until ready to serve.

Cooking Tips

For Deviled Tuna Eggs, substitute one 4-ounce package of albacore tuna for the salmon.

Nutritional Facts

Serving: 1 Half Egg

Calories: 59

Fat: 4 g

Sodium: 92 mg

Total Carbs: 0.6 g

Net Carbs: 0.6 g

Fiber: 0 g

Sugar: 0.6 g

Protein: 5 g

Cooking Conversions

The tables below apply standard U.S. measurements, offering equivalent conversions for United States, metric, and Imperial (U.K.) measurements. The measurements and their equivalents are approximate, and some are rounded to the nearest whole number (source: https://www.nist.gov/pml/weights-and-measures/metric-cooking-resources).

Dry/Weight Measurements

Measure	U.S.	Ounces	Pounds	Metric
1/16 teaspoon	a dash			.25 ml
1/8 teaspoon	a pinch or 6 drops			.5 ml
1/4 teaspoon	15 drops			1 ml
1/2 teaspoon	30 drops			2 ml
1 teaspoon	1/3 tablespoon	1/6 ounce		5 ml
1-1/2 teaspoon	1/2 tablespoon	1/4 ounce		7 grams
3 teaspoons	1 tablespoon	1/2 ounce		14 grams
2 tablespoons	1/8 cup	1 ounce		28 grams
4 tablespoons	1/4 cup	2 ounces		56.7 grams
5 tablespoons plus 1 teaspoon	1/3 cup	2.6 ounces		75.6 grams
8 tablespoons	1/2 cup	4 ounces	1/4 pound	113 grams
10 tablespoons plus 2 teaspoons	2/3 cup	5.2 ounces		151 grams
12 tablespoons	3/4 cup	6 ounces	0.375 pound	170 grams
16 tablespoons	1 cup	8 ounces	.500 or 1/2 pound	225 grams
32 tablespoons	2 cups	16 ounces	1 pound	454 grams
64 tablespoons	4 cups or 1 quart	32 ounces	2 pounds	907 grams

Liquid or Volume Measurements

Jigger	1-1/2 or 1.5 fluid ounces		3 tablespoons	45 ml
1 Cup	8 fluid ounces	1/2 pint	16 tablespoons	237 ml
2 Cups	16 fluid ounces	1 pint	32 tablespoons	474 ml
4 Cups	32 fluid ounces	1 quart	64 tablespoons	946.4 ml
2 Pints	32 fluid ounces	1 quart	4 cups	946 ml
4 Quarts	128 fluid ounces	1 gallon	16 cups	3.785 liters
8 Quarts	256 fluid ounces or one peck	2 gallons	32 cups	7.57 liters
4 Pecks	One bushel			
Dash	Less than 1/4 teaspoon			

Conversions for Baking Ingredients

Ingredients	Ounces	Grams
1 cup of Almond or Coconut Flour	5	142
1 cup of granulated Swerve	7	198
1 cup firmly pack brown Swerve	7	198
1 cup powdered (confectioners) Swerve	4	113
1 cup cocoa powder	3	85
Butter		
4 tablespoons = 1/2 stick = 1/4 cup	2	57
8 tablespoons = 1 stick = 1/2 cup	4	113
16 tablespoons = 2 sticks = 1 cup	8	227

Oven Temperatures

Fahrenheit (degrees)	Celsius	Gas Mark (Imperial)	Description
225	105	1/3	Very cool
250	120	1/2	
275	130	1	Cool
300	150	2	
325	165	3	Very moderate
350	180	4	Moderate
375	190	5	
400	200	6	Moderately hot
425	220	7	Hot
450	230	8	
475	245	9	Very hot
500	260		Broil (U.S.)

For other kitchen conversions, see Convert-me.com.

FREQUENTLY ASKED QUESTIONS

1. What is the keto diet?

The keto diet, short for ketogenic, is a low carb, high fat diet. It is very similar to the Atkins diet, though the Atkins dieters consume more protein than keto dieters. Keto restricts carbs to 20 to 50 grams or less per day, whereas a regular low carb diet considers low carb intake to less than 100 carbs per day.

2. Is the keto diet safe?

Yes, the keto diet is safe. However, those who are on insulin, blood pressure medicine, or breastfeeding need to consult your doctor before you start the keto diet. When consuming a low carb diet, the body's blood sugar reduces.

3. What happens to your body when you cheat on the keto diet?

When following the keto diet, your body changes from burning glucose for fuel to burning stored fat. It depends at what stage of ketosis your body is in when you cheat on your diet. After the body is in ketosis, it doesn't want to switch back to glucose and will give you warning signs such as a slight headache or fatigue.

4. How can I achieve nutritional ketosis?

By consuming no more than 20 to 30 grams of carbs per day, depending on your activity level, you should be in nutritional ketosis after about 7 days. To know if you are in ketosis, test your breath, blood, or urine.

5. How long does it take for the body to get into ketosis?

It depends on your carbohydrate store and your activity. It may take from 2 to 4 days for very active person to 7 to 10 days for a sedentary person.

6. How long should I stay on the keto diet?

Experts say stay on keto for a maximum of six months (Migala 2019). I recommend you reset your metabolism after 12 weeks. However, if you feel you don't need a break or if you are not on a diet plateau, then continue the advance meal plan.

7. Can I drink beer and alcohol while on the keto diet?

Yes, you can; however, the sugar or alcohol content in beer or alcoholic beverages may kick you out of ketosis. It is best to withhold these drinks until you are ready to reset your metabolism. Drink responsibly. Monitor your keto progress and weight.

8. Can I eat bacon while on the keto diet?

Yes. Bacon is considered a main staple in the keto diet because of the good fat you get from the bacon.

9. Do I need to take keto supplements?

No, you don't have to take keto supplements to be on the keto diet. If you want to take a supplement, the MCT oil is a great source for electrolytes and good fat. The BHB supplement is exogenous ketones to help your body attain ketosis or stay in ketosis if too many high carbs are consumed. Be aware if you don't need the exogenous ketones, it can stall your weight loss activity. I also recommend taking a good multivitamin.

10. Will being in ketosis really stop the food cravings?

Yes. If you are in nutritional ketosis, you will not experience food cravings. The cause of most food cravings is the body needing or wanting glucose. Therefore, while you are on glucose, you experience the high and lows of sugar or carbohydrate cravings.

GLOSSARY

The following list of terms and definitions used in this book provides clarity and convenience.

Acetoacetate is the second most dominant ketone enzyme, about 20% of the total ketones in the blood.

Beta-hydroxybutyrate (BHB) is one of three ketone enzymes created by the liver, tallying for 78% of the total ketones in the blood.

Calorie is the quantity of heat required at one atmospheric pressure to increase the temperature of one gram of water by one degree Celsius (about 4.19 joules).

Carbohydrates are various neutral compounds of carbon, hydrogen, and oxygen such as sugars, starches, and celluloses.

Cyclical Keto Diet (CKD) means you're going in and out of keto on a weekly basis. Also known as carb cycling, a cyclical keto diet involves one day a week of carb-loading. The other six days of low-carb keto are identical to the standard keto diet.

Electrolyte is a substance isolating ions and conducting electricity.

Fasting is the self-discipline of not consuming food for a defined period.

Fat is one of three nutrients used as an energy source by the human body.

Fiber is a nutritional material comprising of cellulose, lignin, and pectin elements resilient to the digestive processes.

Glucose is a simple sugar, an important energy source in the human body and a component of many carbohydrates.

High Protein Keto Diet (HPKD) is a modified version where the dieter eats more protein and less fat than the SKD.

Intermittent Fasting is an eating pattern where you cycle between periods of eating and fasting.

Keto flu is collected symptoms such as headaches, nausea, constipation, fatigue, and sugar cravings of the body's withdrawal reaction from glucose and adaption to a ketogenic diet.

Ketoacidosis is a serious complication of diabetes (usually type 1 diabetes) that occurs when the body produces high levels of acids in the blood called ketones, and the body cannot counter by producing enough insulin.

Ketogenesis is a biochemical process organisms produce ketone bodies to break down fatty acids and ketogenic amino acids.

Ketogenic diet is a high fat, low carbohydrates (sugars) diet causing the body to break down fat into molecules called ketones.

Ketones are a chemical substance the human body makes when it lacks sufficient insulin in the blood to produce energy.

Ketosis is a metabolic state categorized by elevated levels of ketones in the blood or tissues because of a low carbohydrate diet.

L-Theanine is an amino acid found most commonly in tea leaves and in small amounts in Bay Bolete mushrooms.

Long Chain Triglyceride (LCT) is a fatty acid containing 20 or more carbon atoms, which are saturated or polyunsaturated fatty acids.

Macros or Macronutrients are molecules from carbs, protein, and fat the body uses to create energy.

Magnesium is an intricate mineral in several processes occurring in the body including nerve signaling, the building of healthy bones, and normal muscle contraction.

Medium Chain Triglyceride (MCT) is a fatty acid containing 6 to 12 carbon atoms. MCTs are generally manmade through the pressing of coconut or palm kernel oils in a laboratory.

Minerals are inorganic elements such as calcium, iron, potassium, sodium, or zinc, essential to the nutrition of humans, animals, and plants.

Nutritional ketosis happens when the human body uses fat instead of glucose as an energy source. The liver converts this fat into chemical elements called ketones and releases them into the bloodstream to burn the ketones as an energy source.

Omega-3 Fatty Acids are an unsaturated fatty acid found in fish oils, especially from salmon and other cold-water fish, containing three double bonds in the hydrocarbon chain.

Probiotics are denoting substance stimulating the growth of microorganisms with beneficial properties in the intestinal tract.

Protein is a group of amino acids, compounds and carbon, hydrogen, oxygen, nitrogen and (occasionally) sulfur found in foods.

Standard Keto Diet (SKD) is a low carbohydrate, high fat diet with similarities to Atkins Diet and other low carbohydrate diets.

Targeted Keto Diet (TKD) is considered an advanced diet approach for athletes, whereas they consume rapid carbohydrates 15 minutes to an hour before an intense workout or competition. The athlete may not consume carbohydrates from fruit during this rapid buildup of carbohydrates.

Triglycerides are a major form of fat stored by the body, consisting of fatty acid three molecules combined with a molecule of the alcohol glycerol and serving as the backbone of many types of lipids (fats).

Turmeric is a bright yellow, fragranced perennial herb powder found in the rhizome of the ginger plant family and used for flavoring, coloring agent or stimulant in Asian and Indian cooking.

Weight Loss Plateau is a temporary stoppage of losing weight when burned calories equals consumed calories (Ciccarelli, 2018).

BIBLIOGRAPHY

Akers, W. (2017, November 02). Keto diet metabolism reset. Retrieved from *Healthline* at https://www.healthline.com/health-news/can-keto-reset-diet-fix-metabolism#1.

Betsch, M. (2015, March 02). 10 Artificial sweeteners and sugar substitutes. Retrieved from *Explore Health* at https://www.health.com/nutrition/10-artificial-sweeteners-and-sugar-substitutes.

Bradley, S. (2018, May 14). What is the metabolic reset diet and can it help you lose weight? Retrieved from *Women's Health Magazine* at https://www.womenshealthmag.com/weight-loss/a20653634/metabolic-reset-diet/.

Buckley, M. (2019, December 27). Free carb counter apps for your low-carb diet. Retrieved from *Hangry Woman* at https://hangrywoman.com/free-carb-counter-apps-for-your-low-carb-diet/.

Ciccarelli, L. (2018, September 18.) Carb cravings? Why you get them (& how to stop them). (Fact checked by Anthony Gustin, DC, MS.) Retrieved from *Perfect Keto* at https://perfectketo.com/carb-cravings/.

Clarke, C. (2019, October 5) How to use intermittent fasting on a keto diet [fasting schedule]. (Medical reviewed by Dr. Barton Jennings). Retrieved from *Ruled.me* at https://www.ruled.me/intermittent-fasting-on-keto-diet/.

Definition of CALORIE. (2020). Retrieved from https://www.merriam-webster.com/dictionary/calorie.

Eenfeldt, A. (2018, June 19). Customize or create your own keto meal plans! Retrieved from *Diet Doctor* at https://www.dietdoctor.com/create-your-own-keto-meal-plan.

Gilson, J. (2018, September 12). How to design your own workout program: a guide for beginners. Retrieved from *Whole Life Challenge* at https://www.wholelifechallenge.com/how-to-design-your-own-workout-program-a-guide-for-beginners/.

Gotter, A. (2017, July 05). Visceral fat. Retrieved from *Healthline.com* at https://www.healthline.com/health/visceral-fat.

Gunnars, K. (2018, January 09). How many carbs should you eat per day to lose weight? Retrieved from *Healthline* at https://www.healthline.com/nutrition/how-many-carbs-per-day-to-lose-weight.

---- (n.d.). 6 health benefits of apple cider vinegar backed by science. Retrieved from *Healthline.com* at https://www.healthline.com/nutrition/6-proven-health-benefits-of-apple-cider-vinegar#section1.

Hendon, L. (2020, October 27). 6 methods to get rid of keto flu for good. Retrieved from *Keto Summit* at https://ketosummit.com/what-is-keto-flu-how-to-cure-keto-flu/.

Herr, L. (2017, May 25). How to set weight-loss goals you can actually achieve. June 5th, 2017, Vol. 189, No. 21, U.S., Retrieved from *EatingWell.com* at https://time.com/magazine/us/4793878/june-5th-2017-vol-189-no-21-u-s/.

Holland, K. (2019, September 18). 15 things you need to know before starting the keto diet. (Medically reviewed by Maureen Namkoong, MS, RD). Retrieved from *The Healthy* at https://www.thehealthy.com/weight-loss/start-keto-diet/.

Janiszewski, P. (2015, December 02). How long can humans survive without food or water? Retrieved from *Medicalxpress.com* at https://medicalxpress.com/news/2015-12-humans-survive-food.html.

Jennings, L. (2020). Food calorimetry: How to measure calories in food. Retrieved from *Carolina Biological Supply Company* at https://www.carolina.com/teacher-resources/Interactive/food-calorimetry+/tr23949.tr.

Kennedy, M. (n.d.). Learning to read labels. Retrieved from *Diabetes Education Online.* Diabetes Teaching Center at the University of California San Francisco at https://dtc.ucsf.edu/living-with-diabetes/diet-and-nutrition/understanding-carbohydrates/counting-carbohydrates/learning-to-read-labels/.

Keto Diet Weight Loss Plateau: How to break it & keeping slimming. (2019, September 25). Retrieved from *Perfect Keto* at https://perfectketo.com/keto-diet-weight-loss-plateau/.

Kossoff, E. (2017, October 01). Ketogenic diet. (Reviewed by Joseph Sirven, MD 2017, October 25). Retrieved from *Epilepsy Foundation* at https://www.epilepsy.com/learn/treating-seizures-and-epilepsy/dietary-therapies/ketogenic-diet.

Kubala, J. (2018, August 21). A keto diet meal plan and menu that can transform your body. Retrieved from *Healthline* at https://www.healthline.com/nutrition/keto-diet-meal-plan-and-menu.

Mawer, R. (2018, August 2). 10 signs and symptoms that you're in ketosis. Retrieved from *Healthline* at https://www.healthline.com/nutrition/10-signs-and-symptoms-of-ketosis.

Migala, J. (2019, January 29). How to maintain your health and weight loss results after the keto diet. Retrieved from *Every Day Health* at https://www.everydayhealth.com/ketogenic-diet/how-keep-weight-off-after-keto-diet/.

Moles. (2019, September 12). Meet the moles! Retrieved from *American Chemical Society* at https://www.acs.org/content/acs/en/education/outreach/moles.html.

Musa-Veloso, K., Likhodii, S., Cunnane, S. (2002). Breath acetone is reliable indicator of ketosis in adults consuming ketogenic meals. *The American Journal of Clinical Nutrition, Volume 76, Issue 1, 65-70.* Retrieved from https://doi.org/10.1093/ajcn/76.1.65.

Oswald, C. (2018, March 22). Digestive enzymes: Amylase, protease, and lipase. Retrieved from *Integrative Therapeutics* at https://www.integrativepro.com/Resources/Integrative-Blog/2018/Digestive-Enzymes-Amylase-Protease-Lipase.

Paoli, A., Bosco, G., Camporesi, E., Mangar, D. (2015, February 02). Ketosis, ketogenic diet and food intake control: a complex relationship. Retrieved from *Frontiers in psychology, 6, 27.* doi:10.3389/ fpsyg.2015.00027 at https://www.ncbi.nlm.nih.gov/pmc/articles/PMC4313585/?tool=pmcentrez&report=abstract.

Phinney, S., Volek, J. (2018, June 06). Ketone supplements: the pros and cons. Retrieved from *Virta Health, Inc.* Blog at https://blog.virtahealth.com/ketone-supplements/.

Rodal, R. (2019, November 13). Cyclical ketogenic diet: Is it right for you? *HVMN.com blog* at https://hvmn.com/blog/keto-diet/cyclical-ketogenic-diet-is-it-right-for-you.

Satterthwaite, L. (2018, December 11). The pros and cons of the keto diet. Retrieved from *ProMedica HealthConnect* at https://promedicahealthconnect.org/wellness/the-pros-and-cons-of-the-keto-diet/.

Shiel, Jr., W. (2018, December 11). Medical definition of carbohydrates. Retrieved from *MedicineNet* at https://www.medicinenet.com/script/main/art.asp?articlekey=15381.

Sifferlin, A. (2017, May 25). The weight loss trap: why your diet isn't working. June 5th, 2017, Vol. 189, No. 21, U.S., Retrieved from *Time Magazine* at https://time.com/magazine/us/4793878/june-5th-2017-vol-189-no-21-u-s/.

Villines, Z. (2019, January 21). Ketosis vs ketoacidosis: Differences, symptoms, and causes. Retrieved from *Medical News Today* at https://www.medicalnewstoday.com/articles/324237.php.

Waehner, P. (2013, August 05). How to properly take body measurements during weight loss. (Reviewed by Tara Laferrara). Retrieved from *Very Well Fit* at https://www.verywellfit.com/how-to-take-your-body-measurements-1231126.

What are normal blood sugar levels? (2018, December 01). (Reviewed by Brunilda Nazario on 2018, December 10) Retrieved from *WebMD* at https://www.webmd.com/diabetes/qa/what-are-normal-blood-sugar-levels.

FURTHER READING

Athletes and Keto

How to be a ketogenic athlete, and what to eat, how to exercise. (2019, November 3). Retrieved from https://www.ditchthecarbs.com/how-to-be-a-ketogenic-athlete/.

Cheating on Diets

Fischer, K. (n.d.). Halle Berry has keto diet cheat days. Retrieved from *Healthline* at https://www.healthline.com/health-news/halle-berry-uses-cheat-days-on-keto-should-you.

Zelman, K. M. (2009, October 22) How to cheat on your diet and still lose weight. Retrieved from *WebMD* at https://www.webmd.com/diet/obesity/features/cheat-on-your-diet-and-still-lose-weight#1.

Cooking Conversions

Grams to tablespoons, and other cooking ingredients conversions. (n.d.). Retrieved from https://www.convert-me.com/en/convert/cooking.

Metric cooking resources. (2019, December 6). Retrieved from https://www.nist.gov/pml/weights-and-measures/metric-cooking-resources.

The Kitchen Whisperer. (n.d.). Retrieved from http://www.thekitchenwhisperer.net.

Diabetes

Diabetic ketoacidosis: Symptoms and causes. (2019, December 11). Retrieved from *Mayo Clinic* at https://www.mayoclinic.org/diseases-conditions/diabetic-ketoacidosis/symptoms-causes/syc-20371551.

Diabetes UK. (n.d.). Know diabetes. fight diabetes. Retrieved from *Diabetes UK*. Retrieved from https://www.diabetes.org.uk/.

Exercise

Can you sing while you work out? (2019, August 6). Retrieved from *Mayo Clinic* at https://www.mayoclinic.org/healthy-lifestyle/fitness/in-depth/exercise-intensity/art-20046887.

Epilepsy

Palmer, C. (2019, March 26). The ketogenic diet may help stop seizures. Retrieved from *Psychology Today* at https://www.psychologytoday.com/us/blog/advancing-psychiatry/201903/the-ketogenic-diet-may-help-stop-seizures.

Fasting

6 keto rules to follow even if you're not actually keto. (2018, June 6). Retrieved from *Women's Health Magazine* at https://www.womenshealthmag.com/health/a21095917/keto-diet-basics-rules/.

The Rules of Intermittent Fasting. (2019, September 22). Retrieved from *Advantage Meal Solutions* at https://www.advantagemeals.com/top-11-intermittent-fasting-rules-for-effortless-weight-loss/.

Food Groups

Clinical Guidelines. (2016, February 5). Low Carb Conferences. Provider Resources. Retrieved from *Low Carb USA* at https://www.lowcarbusa.org/.

Good Fats

Facts about monounsaturated fats: MedlinePlus Medical Encyclopedia. (n.d.). Retrieved from *Medline Plus* at https://medlineplus.gov/ency/patientinstructions/000785.htm.

Facts about polyunsaturated fats: MedlinePlus Medical Encyclopedia. (n.d.). Retrieved from *Medline Plus* at https://medlineplus.gov/ency/patientinstructions/000747.htm.

Reading Nutrition Labels

FM, P. (n.d.). Best Keto Podcasts (2020). Retrieved from https://player.fm/featured/keto.

Tracking Meals and Calories Calculator

Foods. (n.d.). Retrieved from https://www.fatsecret.com/calories-nutrition/.

Recipe Nutrition Calculator. (n.d.). Retrieved from https://www.myfitnesspal.com/recipe/calculator.

Vitamins

Multivitamins Pros and Cons. (2018, September 6). Retrieved from https://best5supplements.com/multivitamins/multivitamins-pros-and-cons/.

Weight Loss

Is Weight Loss on Ketosis Sustainable? (n.d.). Retrieved from https://nutritionfacts.org/video/is-weight-loss-on-ketosis-sustainable/.

YOUTUBE VIDEOS

Arce, M. (2017, February 7). How to do proper measurements for a woman. Retrieved from *Loud Rumor,* YouTube video at https://youtu.be/yFzTzMpqZpA.

Berg, E. (2018, November 11). Dr. Berg's healthy ketogenic diet Basics: Start here. Retrieved from https://youtu.be/vMZfyEy_jpI.

Fat to fit. (n.d.). Retrieved from https://www.youtube.com/channel/UCPgj6A1FAy5zRqfpdFnSw_w.

How to do a keto diet: The complete guide. (2018, December 6). Retrieved from https://youtu.be/sBw2rdwBfZE.

How to make 1carb keto flatbreads - Vegan | Keto. (2018, October 12). Retrieved from https://youtu.be/4MfPzlqguho.

Intermittent fasting. (2019, January 30). Retrieved from https://youtu.be/XeSL_jzMedU.

Keto connect. (n.d.). Retrieved from https://www.youtube.com/channel/UCzRYivTpUQ0r2qPPjfLoQiA

Ketogenic diet: Shred fat & build muscle. (2017, September 19). Retrieved from https://youtu.be/2m3g0JBdtgE.

Keto in Canada. (n.d.). Retrieved from https://www.youtube.com/channel/UC9ED_zKUC_9alLXkprok-8A.

Keto in China: Can you do it? Eating the ketogenic diet in China, low carb in China. (2019, October 30). Retrieved from https://youtu.be/FeJQhDj9irI.

Ketogenic food haul from Aldi UK. (2018, January 14). Retrieved from https://youtu.be/KSF6WUh55cc.

Keto tacos! The ultimate Mexican food! Aye…. (2018, November 9). Retrieved from https://youtu.be/fcaixvq_rIU.

Laura's ketogenic way of life: Australian vlogger. (n.d.). Retrieved from https://www.youtube.com/channel/UC9e8j3_wMm0tifc5qzmhPhA.

Low carb down under. (n.d.). Retrieved from https://www.youtube.com/user/lowcarbdownunder.

Phinney, S. (2018, April 13). Dr. Stephen Phinney on nutritional ketosis and ketogenic diets (Part 1). Retrieved from https://youtu.be/1IEuhp8RFMU.

Tabois, D. (2014, December 12). How to measure your body using a measuring tape. Retrieved from https://youtu.be/3ZSfY87v6pM.

Salvatori, A. (2018, January 11). What to order at a restaurant following the keto diet? Retrieved from Ashley Salvatori at https://youtu.be/D5_lU_5BuXA.

Yummy inspirations. (n.d.). Retrieved from https://www.youtube.com/channel/UCv1rd3I2qtBwtJh0lue2pww/featured.

KETO GROUPS

Many available keto groups exist online. If you perform a search on Google for "Keto Groups to Join," you will receive over 3 million hits.

With these groups, I found Meetup.com, which is a social gathering site for the most part but also contains quite a few Keto Groups or Keto Support Groups. If you proceed to their site at https://www.meetup.com/topics/ketogenic-diet/all/ and type in a particular search topic in your local area such as "Ketogenic Diet Groups to Join in Melbourne, Australia," several groups in your local area will appear in Meetup.

If you know of or if you are a member of a Keto group in your local area, please write me at mikewess@yahoo.com to include it in my second edition printing later. Write in the subject line your Keto group and locale; for examples, "Keto Group in Germany or Keto Group in Denver, CO."

Keto Community Australia. (n.d.). Retrieved from Facebook at https://www.facebook.com/groups/464268613735416/?ref=br_rs.

Ketogenic Diet for Beginners. (n.d.). Retrieved from *Facebook* at https://www.facebook.com/KetogenicDietForBeginners101/.

Ketogenic Diet groups. (n.d.). Retrieved from *Meet Up* at https://www.meetup.com/topics/ketogenic-diet/.

Ketovangelist, L. (n.d.). KetoCon Austin 2020 | KetoCon. Retrieved from https://www.ketocon.org or Contact info at info@ketocon.org or write: 4301 W William Cannon Dr., Suite B150 #524, Austin, Texas 78749-1487.

Low Carb Down Under. (n.d.). Retrieved from https://lowcarbdownunder.com.au/.

THANK YOU

Thank you for reading my book. If you or your loved one found this book helpful, please leave a heartfelt review on Amazon at https://www.amazon.com/dp/B082BG5CPX.

Write me at mike@letsketonow.com or join my community of cooks and readers at https://www.letsketonow.com for more information on the ketogenic lifestyle, recipes, and newsletter.

Best,

Mike

FOLLOW the AUTHOR

Connect with or follow author:

https://www.amazon.com/author/mikewessels

Blog: https://www.letsketonow.com

https://www.pinterest.com/discoverketo/

https://twitter.com/mikewessels5

Join other fans of Discover Your Best Keto Now community by joining the FREE author-led Facebook group: Discover Your Best Keto Now: https://www.facebook.com/groups/172968950657202/

ABOUT THE AUTHOR

Mike is very passionate about his Keto lifestyle and helping others. He enjoys cooking for friends and family. He enjoys learning and writing about everyday life issues to help others.

He lives with his wife, Cindy, and their cat, Jack, in Houston, Texas.

Best wishes and much success on your Keto weight loss journey,

Mike Wessels

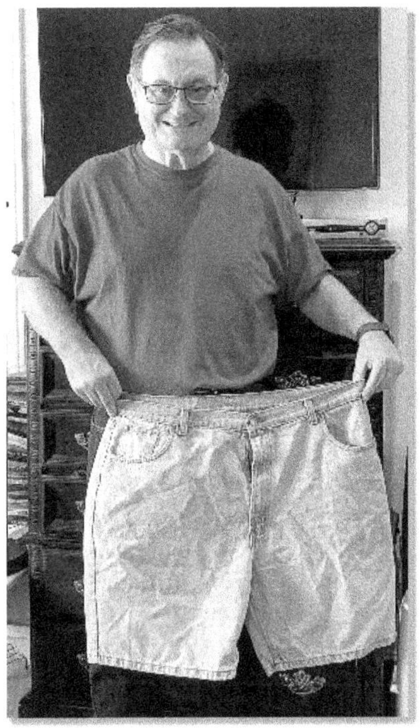